CONTENTS

I dedicate this work to the Great Unknown power, to all masters and teachers of all forms that I encountered in this world and beyond, and to my two children, who helped me see the reason why I should be a better human being.

FOREWORD

I find it so fascinating how life brings people together totally unplanned and how those meetings change our lives forever. This was the story of me and Nicole. We connected in 1993 at a two-week "Healer Heal Thyself" workshop in Trinidad-Tobago that we both attended, along with my husband, Arnie. He is a massage therapist who was a crucial factor in Nicole's path. Arnie and I were immediately drawn to Nicole. She is likable and relatable, with an intuitive and natural healing energy. I had this sense that Nicole was at a critical junction in her life journey. She seemed unsure of her direction, yet she had this strong determination to seek her true self. We bonded instantly as spiritual sisters from a different mother and as healers.

I knew our meeting was a divine intervention and had a profound meaning for our futures. I just started my new path as a healer, transitioning from a nurse specializing in pain and orthopedics to an acupuncture physician and metaphysical holistic health practitioner. As my husband Arnie and I parted our ways, we vowed to remain close, and so we did. We encouraged Nicole to recognize the natural healer within and to stay focused and directed. She first became a licensed massage therapist, the inspiration coming from her many massage sessions with Arnie. Nicole immediately built a reputation of excellence working on many celebrities at an exclusive Fisher Island resort/ spa at Miami Beach.

Not much time passed when Nicole decided to broaden her practice scope by attending school to pursue a doctor of oriental medicine degree. As a stand-out medical practitioner in her field, Nicole's success is attributed to her strengths: knowledge, professionalism, reliability, compassionate empathy, boundless curiosity, a strong desire to learn, and natural healing instincts.

My husband and I have treated a small number of fibromyalgia patients in our practice with limited success. For many healing practitioners, fibromyalgia is a frustrating disease to treat; in fact, many don't even want to take on the disease. I am so proud to say Dr. Nicole has great success in treating fibromyalgia. Her success results from a unique, multifaceted approach not used by traditional medical practitioners. She incorporates diet and nutrition, detoxing, acupuncture, bioresonance, yoga, past-life regression, electromedicine, meditation, deep introspection, organ flushing, and spiritual therapy to unclutter the mind refocus negative thoughts to positive.

Dr. Nicole's book is a remarkable journey into the options that are time tested and true. These options offer hope and a chance to live a full life to her patients. If you found this book, it is by no accident. The universe led you here. This book is a great learning tool for anyone willing to go deeper into their healing by seeking the power of the sages' mind and wisdom. Through these healing methods, you will discover inner strengths by blending spiritual and psychological processes to access and remove self-limitation blocks.

My husband and I experienced exceptional healing from Dr. Nicole's interventions. She immediately zeros in on the root emotional pain stemming from a physical illness manifestation. Her words, thoughts, and voice are so poignant and dead-on. Only an old soul medicine woman could heal as she does. You are never too old to learn something about yourself, which she very delicately points out to you.

I highly recommend this book to my patients with fibromyalgia or chronic pain. There is much to learn about healing the body, mind, and spirit within this body of work. The importance of health on all levels is critical for clarity and understanding. Dr. Nicole delivers a promising, multifaceted approach and perspective to healing a chronic, complicated, and limiting lifelong condition.

We both share the desire to help humanity reach its highest potential. I studied and received a degree in holistic transpersonal psychotherapy as a way of achieving this goal. Imagine living life with joy and happiness that you were born to feel, know, attract, and share with those you love. Imagine mastering your life and living every day with love, joy, peace, and inner harmony.

UNDERSTANDING FIBROMYALGIA

Fibromyalgia (FM) is a medical diagnosis used to define a set of chronic ailments plaguing the sufferers, most of whom are women. It could be a genetic or personality trait or caused by early traumas. The ailments are, generally, widespread feelings of pain and tenderness in localized areas, including joints and muscles; musculoskeletal, neck, and back pain; headaches; insomnia; fatigue; cognitive difficulties; even anxiety and depression.

Fibromyalgia was formerly classified as an inflammatory musculoskeletal disease but is now considered an illness that primarily affects the central nervous system. Fibromyalgia is a complex and debilitating condition that patients fight against. It is studied worldwide by the medical world and scientists, and there is no real cure. As an acupuncturist and Chinese medicine practitioner, I have encountered only six patients plagued by this illness in twenty-one years. Still, any number of people going through pain and fatigue is enough for me to want to ease their suffering.

In wanting to help all of them, I wondered, "besides my massage and acupuncture training, how can I best help them resolve this illness? How could I greatly eliminate their fatigue and remove their pain long enough to feel like their life is normal?" Every case I encountered became deeply personal. I never suffered from this illness. Still, I did suffer another ailment labeled as a "no-cure" autoimmune disease. I conquered it within six months of the diagnosis despite the no cure labeling of my ordeal.

Healers and practitioners of holistic medicines are too familiar because pain is the motivational factor behind why people seek alternative treatments as their conditions worsen and their desire to minimize medication increases. We wish patients would come sooner, when early signs and symptoms start, instead of delaying or waiting for things to get worse. Holistic medicines like acupuncture and Chinese herbal remedy are gentle yet powerful medical tools to manage pain. Unfortunately, the longer you wait, the more difficult and complex it is to help you.

My intention here is not to talk about what is currently known about fibromyalgia but to bring a new awareness to your mind and introduce information perhaps you have never thought of. It's a new paradigm but only to those who were not aware of it. It can be compared to electricity's early discovery in the sixth century by BC. The truth was, and still is, that everything existed within our Universe long ago, and we decided to channel only the information we needed at certain times.

Everything we need to improve ourselves already exists and will be revealed to us as collectively required, in one form or another.

FEAR NOT THE DIAGNOSIS: WORDS AREN'T US

Like the names of many other diseases, the diagnostic word fibromyalgia contains the energy of pain, fear, or panic that could unconsciously affect the sufferer even more. I often hear my patients say, "I have fibromyalgia," or "I have so much pain." This labeling of ourselves every day (silently in our mind or out loud) might put a dent in our well-being. We don't suspect how much impact the power of words has over us. If we could all see or feel the energetic ripple effect words create, I think we would all be so much more careful of how we talk or what we choose to hear day after day.

The way we think of ourselves, in turn, will create the feeling we have about ourselves, and that feeling will build our life based on our thoughts. The ideal scenario could be seeing ourselves as whole and complete first (even if we are sick), acknowledging an unbalance and connection in the biofield, and finally working on all the necessary adjustments. The physical template is something we possess; it is not the only reality about us, and real growth can happen by finding all possible working methods in fine-tuning ourselves.

Presently, and after having worked with my patients diagnosed with this illness, I found fibromyalgia symptoms can be significantly and satisfactorily reduced 80 to 90 percent through various holistic modalities I learned and successfully applied in my practice.

My agenda here in writing this is that I care for people who are suffering all around the world affected by fibromyalgia I experienced an illness with no cure, with almost the exact symptoms of fibromyalgia. Could it be a misdiagnosis? I don't know, but if you put them side by side and compare all the signs and symptoms, only the diagnostic name differs; the suffering is the same. After freeing myself from the clutch of an incurable illness, I understood how I could put my experience to work for someone else. I desire to help shed some light and understand the reasons for your illness from my perspective. There are different possibilities available nowadays to overturn any illness for anyone at any stage of his/her condition.

I have faith in our human capacity to understand beyond all illness complexities and in people who strongly desire to put into something far more exciting and uplifting than just trying to overcome fibromyalgia symptoms with pills and seeing no end to it.

MY PATH TO BECOMING A HEALER

I became a holistic doctor and a traditional Chinese medicine (TCM) practitioner; it was natural. I have a strong healers soul and a heightened sensitivity that has served me well throughout my life and work.

I was born in Vietnam in 1962 during the war. A long and painful journey led me, in 1994, to the United States at the age of thirty. As a child, I was great with my hands and had an inquisitive and observational nature. I wanted to learn everything within my grasp. Feeling and touching people was the first way I discovered the human body and its anatomy. As a child, I spent countless hours looking at and studying my skin, leg muscles, and hands when no one was looking. I was obsessed with studying bodies.

One odd thing that I possessed early on was an awareness of Self, or an invisible Presence in constant communication with me when needed or when I paid attention to it. I thought everyone was like me for a while, having a continuous conversation with that inner Presence. Later on, the feeling became stronger and stronger, but I had no way to know what it was and did not find out until much later in life. This ability led me to feel intensely every person I approached. Every time I laid my hands on people, I could always feel their aches and pains or energetic levels. I consciously have to put a block on it to cease the feelings, but I can also just blend my whole being with my patient and share the divine sense of health within me. I do it with consciousness. We all have innate gifts to share with the world, and I was born with this one.

My desire to make people feel good and relieve pain is intense. Growing up, I was deprived of many essential things that most of us have early in life.

But when we lack on one side, we gain on the other; that's how I see it. I intuitively learned to develop and grow and be in the Presence of Self. This Presence allows me, at all times, to navigate this world of forms that we call the three-dimensional world. With practice, I can now access the fourth and fifth dimensions as well. We all possess this capacity; you just need to tune into it consciously. After I accomplished this for myself, I brought people the gift of touch and healing.

We should give people what we want most for ourselves. In my case, I wanted to feel perfect health, harmony, and peace within; both of those strong desires put me on a quest for a life of challenge.

I had developed a deep connection with my mother. Due to my close association with her, I felt most of her pains. Even though we lived mostly apart, it taught me a lot about human pain and suffering long before becoming a massage therapist. She instructed me on working on her back pain or neck pain when she was sick in my early twenties. I always felt a sense of fulfillment for relieving her of anything painful when I could.

When she became very ill with a cancer diagnosis in 2011, I emotionally and spiritually went through this disease with her, but from a distance. My twin sons, having just been born, the 4,573 miles between us, and how my life was at that time, prevented me from being there for her every day in ways I hoped I could. I knew my lesson here was just to be there in spirit with her and let go of all expectations of healing her. I was to accept whatever was and have perfect faith in her soul design.

Sometimes, we have to accept that healing does not always mean physical healing.

While living in Africa, I spent a lot of time massaging all my friends for no pay. It was a pastime that I later turned into a full professional occupation.

NATURAL PHARMACOPEIA

Our bodies possess the biggest natural pharmacy within. The complexity of how the Innate Intelligence works in repairing is truly beyond our human grasp, and it does a fantastic job. Keeping and improving our health daily is a must to keep everything working and for us to thrive until we exit this mortal frame.

The tips of our fingers are equipped with high-technology sensors and with heightened sensitivity. You can receive or access all energetic information from there. Skin or no skin, we are always exchanging love and affection with consciousness. Deep care for others can be sent across the globe by mere thoughts.

The ability to receive information is not necessarily coming in contact with your physical hand only. Highly sensitive people can receive information from just looking at people, feeling them, and accessing their electromagnetic field. Just through proximity, we can glean a whole idea of their health. New beings of higher consciousness have been coming into existence; we are also receiving further cosmic information. We are updating old files to fit this new awareness of who we are to make sense.

I have learned to detect people's energy, pain, or serious illnesses using my third eye (or inner vision) instead of using my touch. I continually enjoy the connection with and feelings of another as an extension of myself. As I do that, the information allowed for me to receive to help the patient will happen. I do not always have access to a person in this way; sometimes, I have to ask for it consciously.

THE GIFT OF TOUCH

While working as a massage therapist in Fisher Island, there were many instances when an urgent personal fact was "given" to me in a flash. I would speak to the person to consult their doctors or a therapist for emotional issues. That was my early debut working in the healing field. Then, later on, I learned TCM, energetic medicine, and past-life regression therapy. I found these are important and the best adjuncts to my work.

As an empath, I never understood or accepted that someone could feel pain and stress (including myself) and always naturally felt that people were a part of me. At times, feeling a disease is so disturbing to my system that I have to distance myself or block my empathetic nature and close my energetic circuits to perform my work. I can feel pretty sick if I access and stay too long in another person's field. Sometimes, though, I go into the disease, speak to it, channel the messages to find the actual problem, and help the person in front of me.

All that love for touch led me to become a licensed massage therapist first before becoming a physician. My path and my profession in this life were clear to me. My inclination gravitated around health, healing, and making someone feel good. It is true nature to me, no questions asked. Indeed, health is the first important step toward building a strong foundation for our happiness; otherwise, there is no progress toward anything. I always felt the purpose of my birth in this lifetime was to discover how to master that for myself and care for others more efficiently.

This message is a personal one. Parents, it's a great gift to massage your children early on in their life. Your hands have all the love and life medicine they need. A lot of love can be easily transmitted at younger ages. We all are aware that children don't necessarily need more toys or things. They need more touch. Touch is Presence, and Presence is love.

Most adult people I therapeutically engaged through touch are touch starved. If parents massaged their kids more often, there would be fewer unhappy and way healthier adults as their infantile pains would be soothed, recognized, and honored by gifting through touch.

In my earlier days of being an acupuncturist and Chinese medicine practitioner in 2000, I encountered only two or three fibromyalgia cases. Treating all their symptoms did not make sense to me, which left me with more questions than answers. Since the list of complaints was so long, I wondered, "How long is it going to take for my patient to get better? How do I work to eradicate fifteen or more different symptoms going on at the same time in a person?" Yes, I trained to think like a Chinese medicine doctor, and acupuncture does perform well and great, but my inner being pushed me to learn more and go deeper into true healing. Why does someone become sick? What is it we need to "see" to overcome fibromyalgia?

I am stubborn in wanting to help my patients, and as the symptoms to treat were piling up, the pain would move and dance around their bodies. I called that "chasing the healing." I dug in my heels, kept practicing TCM, kept my faith up, and always believed in the deepest part of my being that this problem is solvable.

To be honest, when patients come, we have one hour to "rescue" their body, and that is not enough to get them to perfect health. There are a lot of things to accomplish when assisting a person in healing. One hour is enough to make them feel good, and they come back a week at a time for months (or years). But what happens between when the patient goes home and when they come back for the next visit? Nothing happens. Like acupuncture junkies, I felt they just went for the next "fix me" while being completely asleep to their true healing.

I confess I had to take a deep breath and look within for answers so often because I was not happy to work with my patients in this manner. The truth was that I could relieve their pain, insomnia, and other symptoms, but I felt like I was just patching them. Was I a bad doctor? Perhaps, if seen from that angle. But I still improved their conditions. I made them feel better each time and sent them home only to see them again and again.

I chose to write this book to show what true healing could consist of and explain how to implement it in your daily routine and make it, like eating and sleeping, a continuous plan for a lifetime. Think of this as your life insurance plan. It's like with an IV: drip by drip, you'll slowly take true healing into your body system to transcend and cure your sickness, illness, and disease all by yourself. And if implemented well, it will all vanish one day like a bad dream as it did for me.

REMEMBERING THE GOAL

As our society significantly improves material, technological, comfort, and entertainment levels, our sicknesses take longer to heal and become more sophisticated to understand, more expensive to treat, and more painful to go through for everyone. The more elaborate and comfortable we try to be in the external world, the more pain and sickness happen in our inner being. We involuntarily lost a valuable balance system that was already in place as we went further out on the limb of discovery and creation. Something had to give. Our health was the expense.

We are creating daily from an unconscious basis. We birthed the unwanted, which is taking over. We forgot the true-life direction we are all supposed to be living. When in time did we lose our way? And for what reason?

Creation certainly knew in the "life plan" we would all "lose it" and be sick somehow. Therefore, in its compassion, it ensured we had lots of help available along our way. I have found four great health pillars for us to apply:

heavy-duty medicinal plants for the body, energetic remedies for our energetic templates, a meditation practice for the mind, and prayers for the soul. Simple, isn't it?

When all this happened at first, I was younger and felt very inexperienced to tackle everything. It was intimidating and humbling. But I saw how Chinese medicine could bring solace to many of its symptoms with its beauty and graceful essence. It does not see sickness from the same ideology that Western medicine does.

In TCM, the body is related to the organic ebbs and flow of nature. Chinese practitioner principles deal with yin/yang theory, *qi* (life force), *Shen* (spirit), *Jing* (essence), color, smell, sound, and so on. Indeed, gentle in its approach and with poetic terminology, traditional Chinese medicine is potent when properly administered.

TCM is the result of nature's continuous evolution. It is a compassionate and spiritual medicine. TCM always gave my patients a great healing experience in my years of practice to keep with them. Deep down in my core, coming from a sense of soul duty, I knew I was working against my integrity. I felt I was born a true healer, but my actions and beliefs contradicted themselves. I know that healing has to happen within the person. A resolution of understandings in all forms is needed for the cure to happen.

How I solved health problems and how I should get to the root of why people were suffering became important. I found ways to patiently coach patients. Some responded well to this message, and some preferred to stay in a deep sleep. But I am not judging. It is their calling. I am here to bring permanent solutions to all their problems, but only if they wish me to do so. I came to terms with my methodology. I understood it would be a long and fruitless road at times. The callings are many, but the gate is narrow.

I suspect all doctors and healers know that even with the best intentions, often we just manage people's illnesses. We even use second-guessing treatments at times. It is our livelihood, after all. We conveniently earn our money, and we prefer to stay conventional or go by the book, as society expects us to. But I am not here to be conventional or conformist, nor am I here to perform a duty based on what I see as incomplete truth. I respectfully desire to speak from my soul and from experience to bring light for those who can hear and see.

Why do we have pain among everything else in life? Life seems so unfair when pain is taking over our joie de vivre. When we are in pain, all we can focus on is pain and more pain. Being sick is painful. Growing is painful. Losing is painful. I can go on and on. Take a look around you. Most of us walk in some kind of pain every day. Whatever form the pain in our lives takes, we all have some form of chronic fibromyalgia within us. It's a matter of how many symptoms of fibromyalgia we have. Two? Five? More?

I am a person who rises with challenges like these. Those challenges took me on a long journey to try to understand it all. I searched, went, and drank (literally) from all fountains of knowledge I could find worldwide; dug into my intuitive reservoir; and read from the best masters. I even often asked for heavenly guidance. Whatever it was, my central conviction was that if we have entered this world as a healthy baby (as most of us did – thank God!), then there must be a way to retrace the body's health back to its perfect blueprint, fibromyalgia or not.

My conscience made me aware of this directive to go and experience the healing firsthand. I knew the next thing for me was to open within myself a channel for direction to follow as I went further onto the path of healing myself like no other. We all have something to heal. The moment I acknowledged the desire to learn, all the help I needed to get me there appeared one after another like magic.

As they say, everything takes lots of work, and you must practice before you become an expert at anything. Starting with ourselves is the first step toward healing, and self-realization is the way out of our human misery.

An important lesson learned by me with my fibromyalgia patients is to actualize their truth. They need to be guided to their pain and suffering. If we are willing to tackle a job as difficult as overturning our sickness or disease, it's like reaching a peak for the climber; the task is truly rewarding.

To all people living with fibromyalgia: Are you willing to look at your illness and pain with perfect maturity and have a sincere desire for significant change no matter what? Or are you going to live it on the surface and just let someone else do the work for you or be discouraged because you believe it's genetic? Do you think you have no power over your ailments and bad things just happen to you? If you do, I will do anything to help change that if I can. Something as painful as fibromyalgia that is happening to you right now can also be happening *for* you as a stepping-stone for a greater becoming!

A TRUE OPPORTUNITY

Unbeknownst to you, something better is waiting for you to claim it. The rewards for doing so are unsurpassable, and to my humble knowledge, everyone has their name on it.

For the past six years, I did just that. I entered the world of deep healing, learning about pain and decoding physical, mental, emotional, psychological, and spiritual pain. I spent countless time and energy thinking, deciphering, and meditating. I see all pains as "teachers" that, in turn, wake us up from the slumber of our life. They can be real blessings in disguise if we have not been on pain medication for too long already.

Through my relentless desire to understand authentic healing, I experienced unconventional methods for more meaningful work and an understanding of the nature of sickness and healing. I sincerely think that all diseases, conditions, and illnesses – regardless of whatever names we use for them – have the same root problems. We are all missing the goal here.

When we go off the road, accidents happen. The majority of us are bad drivers of life. The road we were supposed to stay on is narrow and straight, so we all quickly swirl too far right or too far left, missing the destination we are meant to reach. But don't you worry. The Universe is merciful. We all have so many chances. We have a lifetime to go back and try and try and try again.

A FEW STEPS TOWARD WELLNESS

This is a sincere invitation to you to look at the possibility of healing from many sources. Getting to this point in your journey means that you are searching. You are doing the asking and the knocking, and that led you to this simple book.

Just how our huge Universe is at work at all times 24/7, Mother Earth is continuously moving its massive form by rotating on its axis without making a sound. The sun rises and sets every day. Life is continually birthing with a perfect balance enfolded from the stars in the cosmos to the macrocosm and microcosm. It is up to us to follow its example.

Let's admire the perfect mathematics at work for our existence. As unthinkable and unimaginable as it might sound, I can assure you that every minute detail of this planet was carefully thought through, planned for, and cared for. It was crafted to perfection for every species – much like how the chrysalis forms, the caterpillar is born, and the butterfly flies away. Do you think this form of *life* was random? That you do not matter?

Working with yourself only on the physical aspect will give you only temporary relief. Ignoring the more profound universal *truth* can set you back. By knowing your complete ultimate Self, you will enter and acquaint yourself with a realm of divine guidance on the "how" and "what" to heal.

I assure you that the universal truth, carefully thought out, is evident in the many different timelines of your life. Your "eventual" choices bringing you to the present were worked through, helping you get "home and whole" back at the same time. Contrary to how some think, our birth did not occur by sheer luck.

The possibility of enjoying our full existence on earth before we exit this life – the twenty, thirty, or more years we have left in health, bliss, and perfect felicity – is available. I challenge you to realize that your true healthy Self can come forth in this lifetime.

We can work together step-by-step by first taking out the pain and the fatigues. Then, with this set-aside, we can move deeper into psychology and the multidimensional Self we call our perfect Spiritual Being.

STEPS

• Detoxification of the body and getting rid of parasites, fungi, molds, and bacteria. (Required)

• Make better nutritional choices. (Required)

• Find the perfect energetic healing modality to balance your physical body. (Recommended for pains)

• Remove and heal past energetic block patterns, such as traumas, emotional blocks, and negative beliefs that get you stuck. (Required)

• Take on one form of service to give back to society. (Optional but very recommended)

• Choose one exercise that provides deep rest and tranquility. (Recommended)

• Practice meditation as a tool to clear and heal your mind. (Highly recommended)

• Determine which unconventional remedies are available.

DO THE WORK

You are powerful. It is empowering to realize that you are the real doer and maker of your healing. Isn't it so?

ADOPT A NEW MENTAL ATTITUDE

You are the change you want in your life. It is excellent advice to stop procrastinating, to stop blaming others for our unhappiness, and to stop looking on the outside for monetary or temporal excuses. You possess a brain and a will to execute all choices in your life. Fear may stop you or slow you down, but it is only coming from a busy, despotic mind. Nip it in the bud.

Inviting and acknowledging your Higher Being to be with you at every step of the way should be the first thing you do every morning before getting up.

THINK OUTSIDE OF THE BOX

Some of my techniques proposed might be utterly foreign to you. Keep an open mind to explore new things. As you step into the unknown, lots of good things will happen, and it doesn't matter if they do not make sense to you now. They will come later on. Because you dare to ask, knock, and try harder, the Universe will instantly respond. Your healing process will naturally happen. Have faith.

KNOW AND TRUST THAT YOU ARE HEARD

If you don't see the "God," it does not mean it does not exist. "What does the God/ Universe have to do with fibromyalgia?" you ask. I will answer honestly from my experience: everything. If God created man and man created disease, it is obvious we must go to the Creator for help. Wisdom calls us to go to the source to fix the problem.

Let's look at our own body and see how intricate and sophisticated it is and how connected it should be with its Creator. Rest assured, it knows everything about you.

KNOW THIS HIGHER BEING IN YOURSELF (GET ACQUAINTED WITH IT)

I am not referring to intellectual knowledge, such as knowing the encyclopedia by heart. I might have a great memory, but that certainly does not make me intelligent. To *know* deeply is the same as *being*. It's a state of pure Presence within you that is alive at all times and is never separate from you. If you channel this innate supreme power within your Self, it will take center stage in your life, and you will be on your way to greatness. Sick or not, you won't care anymore. This truth will free you from all sufferings, big or small.

DEVELOP YOUR INTERNAL DIVINE COMPASS FOR GUIDANCE

There are so many different holistic modalities out there for this kind of work. It can be overwhelming to navigate them all, but you can find what suits your needs or what is in perfect resonance with you. I invite you to experience as many as possible.

Some tasks will demand your time and money; others need strength, courage, patience, faith, and endurance. We know that nothing of quality comes easy, and the mind always goes for what is familiar, cheap, quick, easy, and painless. The time needed to get to a better place health-wise depends on you. Patience and persistence are key factors, and it will take the time that's necessary – no more, no less.

Your expectations might be too high or want to go too fast, and you could run into disappointments if they are. Go through the journey of self-discovery, keep your eye on the goal of healing and health, and relinquish from your mind expectations of timing. If you don't, you might miss the real purpose.

WHO ARE WE AND WHY ARE WE HERE?

"To think health when surrounded by the appearances of disease, or to think riches when in the midst of appearances of poverty, requires power, but he who acquires this power becomes a Master Mind. He can conquer fate. He can have what he wants.

This power can only be acquired by getting hold of the basic fact which is behind all appearances, and that fact is that there is one 'Thinking Substance,' from which and by which all things are made. Do not ask why these things are true, nor speculate as to how they can be true; simply take them on trust. The science of happiness begins with the absolute acceptance of this faith."

— WALLACE D. WATTLES

This chapter explains the concept that we are energetic beings and that the body is the result of this energetic field; learning to disengage from the body to fully embody our spiritual template allows us to step into another dimension of consciousness where all the possibilities of healing reside.

YOU ARE ENERGY

In *truth*, you are not a body – your body is only an extension of yourself. And you are certainly not the sickness either. Who are you then? You are a boundless field energy experiencing this life with a body. Your energetic field is broken, disrupted with leaks and holes, with a dark and murky pattern in it – and perhaps has been this way for many lifetimes. If this sounds foreign to you, I understand. It's been proven scientifically that everything in or around us is filled with energy. Even Einstein talked about it – I am sure you know him. Even nothingness is energy. If you can shift a part of your mind in accepting this truth, it will be easier to meditate and see and feel the true Presence in action at all times.

You can also feel that energy from your own hands if you try to sense your palms at two or three inches apart. When my acupuncture studies took me to China to expand my learning, I went to the mountains in Shanghai, where I studied for three weeks at a Chinese hospital that combined Western medicine with *qigong* (Life Strength). The group I traveled with was there to learn how to feel energy forms from nature and to practice *qigong* three hours or more a day. I could not put my hands down. For a deep and sensitive person, it was an amazing experience. I felt the trees, plants, flowers, shrubs, and even grass. It was a different feeling; each and everything has its energy signature.

Your body is also a hologram of something much bigger. I don't want to scare you by saying we are not really "real" or that we are only temporarily during this time in our bodies. Just like a movie, our whole life is projected upon a screen. We are actors in that movie. What kind of movie would you like to create? How about becoming the producer of that life movie of ours, if we so choose?

It takes training to feel. We live in a world of the five senses; therefore, we have lost our ability to truly feel because the feeling (besides our emotions of sadness, anger, and joy) was cut off for protection. We don't want to feel pain; therefore, we learned to close this higher sense. Now, our ability to feel, sense, be psychic (like for animals), and see danger is lost, but we can all learn to regain this lost ability to sense.

From difficult circumstances, I grew up and lived feeling my life around. When I was in my survival mode, it helped me avert danger or read people's intentions. I thought everyone could do it. I developed a deep sixth sense or intuition. Sometimes, while I was treating a person, a piece of information was presented to me from nowhere. I did not look for it; it just happened. When I must know specific information about a patient for her betterment, I will know it. Sometimes I share it with the patient, and other times I don't until the patient is ready.

I feel from my third eye most of the time; therefore, I developed a deep vision or intuition of everything around me. Feeling from the heart center possesses another kind of feeling. It is more expansive, peaceful, and blissful. It's a higher frequency. From there, you can feel unity, love, and compassion for all forms. With an elevated sense, we can detect a spiritual and vibrational fragrance.

I remember a picture hung on the abbey wall where I lived from my Catholic upbringing, showing him with his finger pointed to his heart. I questioned this picture for a long time. Later on, while I was studying and practicing chakra (energetic spiritual centers) meditation, the lesson dawned on me like a flash, and I understood the magnificence of the heart center and the third eye. Our bodies' communication needs to be activated and cultivated for our lives to move ceaselessly and effortlessly while carried by those energetic centers called chakras. In English terms, it's like seven active energy reservoirs that go undiminished. If we can tap into them, they will propel us toward growth and empower us in every aspect of our lives. It's an energetic spiritual blueprint we possess throughout our life. Due to ignorance, its real power is absent for most people, as it is not acknowledged in the West.

We can look at suffering from fibromyalgia as a "bad" thing, but in truth, because we are not just a body, nothing is totally negative, and nothing is totally positive. We can only judge from a body/mind perspective something we possess right now; if we were only energy in motion, we would not have this option to consider. Every situation in life can be appreciated from both angles. Things are neither good nor bad – they just are. Observing and assessing constant changes happening around us (like the seasons) and becoming an unmoved observer with no judgment in mind lets us appreciate the scenery of our life.

Being nonreactive does not make us insensitive, just detached. And in doing that, I find we are certainly more proficient because the negative emotion does not get in the way, and we can assess the problem from a more objective place.

Once we know that we are an energy source, our attention can easily (with practice) shift from a life of suffering to a higher truth and understanding. What we focus on takes form. With a deep focus on that energetic field (the Presence), we will grow into something bigger. That enormous Presence will expand exponentially from within us.

Energy has a frequency. I'm not a quantum physicist, but I can explain that energy is a wave measured in frequency. The greater the energy, the larger the frequency is. When you are depressed and sick, your energy level is low; therefore, the frequency is small, and the protection (energetic field) around the body does not work well. It shrinks in size and becomes weak; your aura weakens, and you attract all kinds of diverse problems. A weak energetic field can attract hosts of unwanted parasitic entities, viruses, and anything similar to that frequency level. Every "blow" can penetrate the body, first, energetically, and then move physically and emotionally. By strengthening this energetic shield in and around us with repetitive mental exercises, we can positively impact our energy body's health and create a form of external protection.

We do energetic work to enhance and complete the healing and growing process of our whole being. Our body is a multidimensional being. Healing only the body does not make sense because we miss the bigger picture that needs to become the ultimate being that we were programmed to become.

Perhaps you have been suffering for a long time with fibromyalgia, and you focus on the pain and fatigue all day and night. If you have insomnia, this can drive you to silent despair. Financially, you might be in a bind. Your relationships might suck too. Besides the ill feelings and emotions to overcome and a long list of what doesn't work in your life right now, all you are experiencing is a lot to deal with. It can drive you to want to ignore it all. As we are not feeling good, worse things start to be attracted to us like a magnet – that is the work of frequency going down on you. But we can learn to go up instantly; as we mature spiritually, we develop higher consciousness, which can be beneficial in attracting better things to us.

Most of us learn to accept and cope with whatever is happening quietly. Nope! Don't do that. I would face the bull like a real matador if I were you. For true life to happen and flow, it is imperative to go to your existence's root events and deal with them. I don't know all of your present conditions, and I agree with Socrates: "All I know is I know nothing." But one thing I've known since birth is that we did not come here to live in pain and suffer needlessly. Whether the pain is emotional, physical, or spiritual, there is a way *out* of that. What's the reason to be here otherwise? When we are sick, nothing tastes good.

When utilizing conventional medicines to cure chronic issues, it seems the more we try to "fix" our sickness, the more toxic our body becomes. That leaves most people discouraged, and they end up accepting life as it is because it is the only reality presented to them. If consistently and wrongly guided, dealing with something as fragile and elusive as health in a world of surgery and medicines just worsens the outcome. We could easily miss the potential for growth with a body burdened with the wrong medications.

Happiness here on third-density Earth is illusory and transient. It can show up one day and disappear the next. All the "goodies" of life and the elevated emotions we all want are (most of the time) emulated by external stimuli of wants and desires. No wonder happiness is not a permanent state of being. All we do is cope until finding the next fix to give that feeling of "wow" to our life. What we want is to establish some forms of permanent health and happiness.

We want something that does not fluctuate at the drop of a hat or depends on external conditions. Do you know we all possess a hidden power waiting to be harnessed, ready to be discovered, and available to us for use at all times and places? It exists, and it's called God or supreme consciousness.

Does it sound too unreachable to you? Well, let's make it even more far-fetched then. In truth, we are beings of supreme beauty and power, but we left our real home (once upon a time in the cosmic Universe). We, as God's children, challenged ourselves – "Oh, how fun would it be if we covered ourselves with a cloak of deep ignorance and total forgetfulness to be utterly lost and then find our way back home?" We hid our brilliance and oneness with God so well, went to play down here on earth, and got stuck in the illusion of dense materiality with a physical body we believe is our own. The thick crust covering our divine identity overtook our spiritual intelligence. Now, we find ourselves locked up in a dungeon that's impossible to escape. It's called the mind, and *voilà!* We are stuck in time and inside a human body that ages and gets sick. Yikes! The rest belongs to science fiction.

Let's not perpetuate the belief that we are purely just a body by ignoring the natural gift of our true nature or by procrastinating and being too lazy to think for ourselves. Yes, we are mighty spiritual warriors burdened only by an egoic mind devoid of pure wisdom! The sickness we experience was never ours to own forever; it's only a catalyst for change! We all possess an un-awakened God-given nature. It is not perceivable to most, but if we choose to stir ourselves out of this deep trance, we can be so transformed and rise above an average existence.

The three-dimensional world of what we can perceive with our two eyes is an illusion with mirrors and chimes hanging all over the place. We are like moths flying too close to the flame. Children of spirit can consciously reclaim our true divine inheritance by learning to tame the mind and understand how to eradicate the ego when necessary.

What on earth do we need to do in this life that could be meaningful in terms of "healing ourselves" and reaching for a life of supreme happiness all together? Is being born, going to college, getting a career, getting married, having kids, and growing and dying in sickness the only program available for us to live with?

Tell me, besides obvious bodily self-gratification, when have you ever been genuinely high in happiness by yourself just sitting with nothing or no one? Try this: sit quietly, close your eyes, and tell yourself, "I am so pleased and fulfilled in every aspect of my life, and I trust that all is perfectly well." Using kinesiology, test yourself for an answer. Just feel your response. How true does this ring to you?

Meet the challenge to realize your deepest Self with courage, determination, and focus on going through the work and solving a fascinating enigma. Our Lower Self is inclined to live by ignorance, which causes the great divide between you and your divine nature. Many people believe they have to change the world; the only one to change is genuinely themselves. The world need not change. It's perfect as it is, in my humble belief.

Changing ourselves – that alone is the divine purpose of our life missed by many up until now. This kind of work requires time, patience, and dedicated perseverance. One lifetime is hardly enough due to a distracted mind – hence, reincarnation. We understand why some people go to the mountain in a far distant place to perform the task of self-realization. But from my perspective, we don't have to. We can do it anywhere at any time; it's available for anyone.

Life is medicine itself. We can use each instance of our lives as an opportunity to pursue the realization of our super being, exactly where we are. There is no need to go anywhere – even though I did that. If you have time and money, you like traveling, and COVID-19 is not an issue, you are welcome to travel. There are tons of treasures to experience in this world. But all that is not necessary. Mother Universe procures the same opportunity to accomplish the *work* for all. Why crumble under a life of difficulties and struggle while sitting next to your supreme Self, oblivious to your power at hand? Why go to your tomb one day (sooner than you think) and not be acquainted with who you might be? It is above and beyond all limited knowledge that we possess. Give it a real try. The proof is in the pudding.

We can be the ordinary human who repeats and repeats the cycle of life and death, believing in an illusory existence in which we never have any power. If you decide to pursue finding your God Self within, make sure it is ecstatic and coming from an unshakably strong desire to get there; don't give up. God or Universe does not respond well to lukewarm minds seared in doubts. A mind in a surviving mode always goes to dark and gloomy; it is suspicious. Most of the time, because its job is to "protect" the egoic being (the personality), it always takes a fear-based tactic; it will take you to the no man's land of despotic creation, which, in turn, has no end and no growth.

There is a proverb that says, "What you resist, persists." You resist the sickness, and the illness persists. You fight pain and suffering, and they continue. The mind keeps creating your apparent thoughts. In this case, what is it we are creating? Fear? Sickness? Poverty?

Presently, your body needs attention and TLC. Reverse the current by talking to and loving your painful symptoms as if, like the energy that came and will depart soon. Pain is just a warning signal that forces your attention and redirects and stirs your doings, mind, and spirit in the right direction. *Relax* and *accept* what *is*. You can be in control.

To receive insights, learn to detach yourself from the problem mentally. Create some space between *you* and the situation. The body is just a vehicle. Whatever your question is in your quest to heal, your powerful Self will reach out to let you know the way.

Assess your health and life; assess what needs to be done without judgment, and then calmly accept where you are right now health-wise. There is nothing intrinsically "wrong" with you; in truth, you can never go wrong. It's a "mechanical problem" you must handle, and you can fix everything given the right tool.

The physical body is a hologram existing in this third density. Now, if you decide, you can step into another dimension to gain a better, more objective perspective. I am asking you to widen the windows of cosmic perception. If there is a stumbling block like sickness, clip it in the back of your mind for a little while, drop the analytical mind, bring the consciousness to your heart, and try to feel your "I Presence" (God Self within). As soon as you start the feeling process, go with your mind two to three feet outside your body. It's an exercise that will teach you to reach outside your own body's boundary to feel its vastness.

Once you can spot your own I Presence at will, you can always consciously bring up that awareness. It will carry you upward in its higher-vibratory frequency every day, and the feeling of anything low will just disappear like magic. The negative mind will not have any power over you; it will free you all together.

Nothing is impossible in this world. We can go ahead and nurture this kind of thinking and become limitless creators. This chapter is important because it conveys something so intangible yet so powerful for you to grasp. It is a pivotal work that will help you understand how to transform from a helpless human to breathing, living human dwelling with God.

Let's remove blocks from the body by first checking our belief system/childhood traumas and learning how to *eliminate them from our subconscious*. To remove self-denigrating and limit beliefs imposed on us from cultural, parental, and societal programming, we must start promptly and assess everything about ourselves as thoroughly as possible. Dissect your life like a skilled surgeon and shake everything up. Leave no piece of sand that can stop "the big clock" from working correctly.

It can take a while if you are accepting and sincerely doing it. The time to get there should not be a deterrent to your effort. On the subconscious level of work, you should have professional help to speed up the healing process: hypnotherapy, past-life regression, and psychedelics (which may not be for everyone but are recommended highly).

The journey to Self can be overwhelming sometimes; to do it all by yourself is impossible. The older we get, the more crap we carry within us. At times, we need potent remedies to do the job.

Our hypnotic past, especially during our earlier years, created all our present behaviors, what we choose, and why we choose the things we do. We run through our days on autopilot instead of being conscious of our actions. Healing the past hypnotic behavior based on traumas, negative beliefs, and even past lives can set you on your real journey. You can be free to create the exact life you want beyond any limitation imposed by this three-dimensional reality.

Do the "shadow work" diligently and get deeply personal with yourself. Dig and weed out what makes your body and mind so sick. What happened in your thought process growing up that crippled your perfect blueprint? For too long, we let the world happen to us unwillingly. The time has come to awaken. The energy is available to us right now. Something so unique is occurring right now in our Universe. The possibility to awaken is within reach of those who choose to listen and rise above a conditioned existence that has been perpetuated for too long.

Many great holistic doctors and thinkers in the past offered healing solutions. They also knew and understood the "problem" of negative emotions as energy stored in our body's cell memories. Take it out.

I learned a lot from Dr. Edward Bach, who created the Bach Flower Remedy; Dr. Samuel Hahnemann, who invented homeopathy; Dr. Edgar Cayce wrote *The Sleeping Prophet*; Raymond Rife, an American scientist; and many more. They all launched revolutionary ways of healing the body and mind without harmful chemicals.

I spent six years working through all my emotions, memory cells, and ancestral memories embedded in my genetics. From the moment I felt something was not quite right in my world, I knew my everyday quest was, "How do I free myself from a life of 'bondage' and servitude to the mind?" Because this mind of mine made me suffer in ways no one else was, and I did that to myself.

There is nothing to deny from within ourselves. Our emotions are to be understood and set free. Let them flow like a stream: unimpeded and fluid. Don't hold back this flow – the stream, like energy, needs an unimpeded course.

Clearing out all clutter and freeing your mind is crucial work. I don't know of a more challenging work than this. I did it myself. It is a miniature death occurring again and again – the death of the egoic identity known as the mind.

Most people live by acting and reacting to events and situations, often negatively triggered by those deep beliefs and traumas. They are never truly aware of what caused it in the first place. They never feel genuinely alive because deep garbage removal has to take place first to feel the true life within us truly. Clean that house. The soreness and pain could have been there for eons, lifetimes after lifetimes, crystalized and fossilized into their energetic field and acting out through the body as aches, pains, sicknesses, and diseases.

We are suffering from our inability to feel our deepest Self, our true Self, our God Self. That's all it is. The body is devoid of its true beauty and intelligence. Therefore, true healing needs to happen because our deeply ingrained belief that we are just a body completely disconnects us from the authentic Source energy capable of performing the magic of perfect healing in you.

To make matters worse, we don't even have a clue about our true identities. The "bad" stuff, such as death, suffering, and sickness, will eventually surface and bring up all the more profound layers for us to deal with one day soon enough. The work we can perform to get better could be seen as a hard-earned, personal, and deliberate effort, given its impossible nature at times. And before we let go and let God, there is this mind to fix first.

I say, "Let's *do the work!*"

5

WHAT MAKES US SICK

"We have to awaken to our past, and then, we can set a course toward a meaningful future…"

— TERRENCE MCKENNA

In this chapter, I introduce to you concepts of what causes us to get sick. Understanding this vital chapter can spark your desire to get well no matter how complex you feel.

CASE 1

Helene, my patient, diagnosed with fibromyalgia, came one-day complaining of debilitating fatigue and spent her life lying on the sofa. She had problems with focus, joint pain, lower back pain, neck pain, a constantly sore throat, headaches, brain fog, memory lapse, psoriasis, arthritis, and more. Her energy level was at 20 percent. She told me how the fatigue left her with no strength to do anything, and her legs felt like they could not support her body. She spent the majority of her time sleeping and not doing anything during the day.

The energetic scan I used showed many heavy metals in her immune system and brain tissue. Her thyroid and immune system reading was way low, which indicated highly toxic heavy metals inhibiting everything in her body from functioning normally. The high number of toxic metals lowered her immune system, putting her at increased risk for many forms of infection.

I ordered for her to do a complete total body detox right away. She was compliant in changing and improving her diet as well. In two weeks, her energy level went from a two to an eight on a scale of ten. She received acupuncture; energetic frequency therapy; detoxification of all heavy metals, parasites, fungus, and mold removal; supplements; correct nutrition information; and infrared sauna treatments.

Today, she lives a normal life and is happy about the dramatically quick turnover and positive results she received within three to four weeks. She is naturally inclined to do spiritual work independently, such as meditation, which dramatically helps her stress levels and peace of mind. She adopted better nutrition habits and healthier cleaning products to use in her home. Now, she is independently doing her healing when needed and does not require my help in her recovery. She learned a lot from my advice. I'm so proud of her.

CASE 2

Another patient with fibromyalgia came to my office complaining of extreme fatigue and pain all over her body. The fatigue was high and constant. I had been treating her, and her health was stable. It had been months, and I had not seen her. After her intake, I asked her if she did something different that triggered intense fatigue. After a moment of thinking, she told me that three days earlier, she decided to clean her entire bathroom with Clorox products, and that's when her energy went out the window. I provided the Sensitiv Imago treatment and put her on the Rife machine. Her strength came back, and her pains subsided significantly. She reported that she was able to sleep and got back on her feet the morning after.

The energetic scan showed high amounts of toxic fumes in her system again, and her lungs and brain were significantly affected by them. It all made sense to me: her sensitive systems were not putting up with her cleaning that bathroom for hours and breathing toxic fumes from regular cleaning products. After that incident, she decided only to use cleaning products made with natural and safe materials.

You might not feel that bad when using regular cleaning products if you think they were never a problem. I ask you to think twice. Ignoring or not seeing the problem does not mean it's not there. Toxic heavy metals and cleaning products we use in our everyday life accumulate for years and lower our immune system, causing insurmountable health problems later. They penetrate the skin and invade brain tissue, the lymphatic system, organs, etc. I don't need to go any further for you to see how our insidious, toxic world is a big part of our health problems. All we can do is detox frequently and rebuild and regenerate with holistic and personal healthcare.

I treat house technicians and manicurists as patients too. All were developing skin problems, such as vitiligo and lung cysts. They spent most of their young adult life working in daily contact with highly toxic products such as chlorine and breathing in a highly toxic environment. We absorb lots of toxicities, especially when they are in touch with our skin.

In traditional Chinese medicines, lungs and skin are two organs working together. Lungs problems will show on the skin after some time.

DOING THE WORK BY DIGGING FOR BELIEF PROGRAMMING AND HEALING TRAUMAS

Start from the beginning. Dig into the past and ask yourself all these questions.

How was your childhood? How were your parents with you? Were you happy growing up? Did any major physical/emotional trauma or abuse happen in your life? Are you a perfectionist or a hoarder? Do you like to be in control? Do you have a hard time recognizing or accepting your mistakes? The list of questions to ask yourself will be revealed to you as you go inward to dig out your feelings toward your past.

Answer all questions and check all the possibilities within yourself that can hinder your happiness as an adult now. Is there anything unpleasant and repetitive, such as feeling unworthy, shameful, or guilty, or lacking self-confidence? Do you keep attracting the same toxic relationships that drive you toward your negative feelings? Do you have no power or control over them? Those are like seeds that will be a source of negativity buried inside you, living in your body's cell memories and manifesting as sickness if left and not resolved. They become stuck negative-energy cysts.

This process is self-inquiry. Spending a lot of time with yourself is paramount to finding out what does not serve you right now and why your life feels stuck. "What makes me sick today?" is the right question. It is one major step to weed out all stuck emotions. We act and react based on the values we received growing up.

The false personality births itself as a second shield to camouflage and protects children who cannot relate to a confusing adult world. The beauty of their innocence is lost behind the chain of dramatic events caused by unconscious parenting. Too often, the child in us finds himself/herself with no outlet to freely express his/her highest emotion.

Violence, anger, confusion – these unprocessed emotions will be directed inward because children do not know how to manage them. It is imperative to recognize, heal, and transmute them ASAP.

If you don't remember anything of your life growing up, it is undoubtedly due to being young. You were "asleep" most of the time – we all were. Children use a natural form of automatic protection to cope with the world around them to survive. Awareness was not fully activated then; therefore, consciously, you can't remember it all. But your body and subconscious record and remember everything, and you can tap into them to retrieve valuable information and discard what isn't needed.

This kind of work requires attention and control. There are therapies we can attend and learn through seminars: emotion-focused therapy, PSYCH-K, body talk, cranial-sacral therapy, phoenix rising therapy, Feldenkrais Method, Theta Healing, hypnotherapy, past-life regression therapy, and much more.

UNDERSTANDING KARMA

In the world of physics, we can connect the dots with three phrases: "What we sew, we shall reap," "Do unto others as you would have them do unto you," and "For every action, there is an equal and opposite reaction."

That is karma. It's of our conscious making, not a punishment from above. Anybody in the pursuit of enlightenment or health and his/her right mind will think twice before doing an illicit action and will learn to control his/her mind at all times for positive thoughts toward everything happening around him/her. Thoughts carry weights to be realized in the physical world.

Thinking of or wishing for something that is not for the well-being of ourselves and others will deny our life of its many blessings. It is much easier than we think and more beneficial for our life and our surroundings. Our entire existence is birthed from the law of reciprocity. Lower vibrational thought patterns create pockets of energy, blocking the higher consciousness from reaching us. Our spiritual template becomes discordant and compromised for higher work and will deteriorate.

Hence, it is crucial to learn to control the reactive mind and discordant thoughts. Thoughts are essential – action is carried out based on those. Anything we continuously think, whether consciously or unconsciously, becomes our truth to be lived and experienced. Nothing is lost in this reality or forgotten. We are magicians carrying the power to manifest the highest impossibility, changing lead into gold like skilled alchemists.

Studies show that humans have more than six thousand thoughts per day! If all you think about is your money problems, that can solidify anything quickly in the theme of manifestation.

To master our thoughts is to master our karmic life. It occurs every second of our life, like a powerful magnet that attracts pleasant or unpleasant situations, health, or sicknesses. Thoughts are going around the world like powerful energetic lines attracting their counterparts and setting into motion its realization to reach the thinker.

The more we focus on something, the more it is attracted to us. My deceased mother was so obsessed about her apartment being robbed in Paris in Rue Ernestine, and sure enough, she was robbed during the daytime.

I proposed a simple solution: *relax*, be aware and present, accept. Let the uncontrolled things that need to happen, happen. Let it all go and gracefully bow to the perfect design of this Universe. We are constantly walking to our death bed every day. We need to just surrender to *what is* and concentrate on doing the *work* at hand to elevate the vibrational frequency of our thoughts.

Karma happens every second, but if we earnestly tackle and beautify our inner Self every day, our karma load will lighten up and be significantly diminished. We can pulverize it all with our positive karma. The deliberate positive creation ensued from our own making and effort – in this case, our thoughts – can later allow better outcomes for our health and our mental well-being to be birthed and experienced.

Karma is not necessarily something that accrues from one lifetime to another. It is happening at every moment, like the ticking of a clock or the coming and going of waves crashing on the rocks. It creates a block that separates God's deep inherent connection, which should be as natural to us as breathing.

Remedy

For years (besides meditation), my daily exercise is to repeat a short prayer continually in my mind. We can call it the mantra repetition or *Japa*. A mantra is composed of sacred sounds that someone repeats silently or out loud to keep the mind from wandering. The mind learns to go back to this sound, like the needle of a compass returning to true north.

If you are familiar with mantras, then chanting *"Om Namah Shivaya"* is the most powerful one, according to the Living Avatar Babaji of the Himalayas (he means a lot to me). It means, "I bow to the Consciousness of Infinite Goodness," which is God. As far as I am concerned, we can never go wrong with this one.

Everyone should choose a mantra of their own. It could be in English or any other language. It could be something you say that means you put the Universal Consciousness, God, or something bigger and greater than yourself above all. The goal here is not to obsess with a world of problems but to firmly fix your mind with the name of creation.

In time, the mind will give in to this inner repetition of prayers, and the thought energy emanating from it will neutralize, slow down, and stop the unwanted karmic loops. If you keep doing it, you will master your thoughts and step into creating a higher mind. But until then, keep doing it. Don't worry about anything: *that* which you persistently think shall grow more and more each day and will provide your life with more ease and bliss and bless you with everything you so desire. Saying it out loud is also recommended to prevent the mind from wandering and keeping you stuck in the thoughts that make you sick. The repetitions of the name of God is like a meditation in action. It's a powerful remedy for our monkey mind.

For people on the path of arduous spiritual search already, being initiated to a mantra by a perfected master would be a tremendous help as it connects and ignites the dormant spiritual energy residing in your heart.

Like everyone in life, I experienced tumultuous thoughts and disturbing situations, and I could feel my mind was taking me down too many times. Realizing I could stop my mind from harming me, I said this mantra chant out loud with my feet steeped in water to enhance the magnetic body's cleansing. After chanting my mantra ten thousand times (it's pretty fast, actually), I always emerged thoroughly cleansed, recharged, and detached from the problem or its negativity. It is a powerful weapon to redirect our minds. The frequency of a mantra is of a higher vibration, and it is not just for spiritual benefits but also psychological/ physiological healing. After many years of practicing *Japa*, my mind automatically tunes in my mantra without effort. My life is relieved from me manifesting things I did not want to happen. It now attracts things that I want.

The world will always be what we think it is. So, how do we see this world? If we cannot understand this "world" we live in, why not the go-to source for its real understanding? The world of minds is alluring and unavoidable. Everything is created from mind-stuff that is going on endlessly. Going with one thought only will save us tons of energy, so we don't dissipate and waste powerful energy used to create miracles in our own lives.

MIASM (CHRONIC DISEASES)

A *miasm* can be seen as obsolete to certain schools of thought, but it is as real as *qi* in acupuncture or traditional Chinese medicine. It is relevant for specific modalities but may not be for others. However, in my experience, miasm is seen as a distortion in a person's energetic field. It is essential to understand that what we cannot see can often disturb our health.

The word "miasm" means "vibrational dissonance." Miasms tend to deplete and corrupt the individual's energetic blueprint, which distorts the personal field template he/she is operating. Therefore, the information getting to the person (the physical template) will not be accurate. The awareness of free choice will not be made clear, and the essence of understanding divine *truth* will be significantly reduced by bad karma. There is a build-up of miasms from personal to collective, through your family DNA and ancestors for many generations. It's called the karmic imprint, which is holographically projected into our body, mind, and three-dimensional life experiences through the natural law of multidimensional manifestation. "What you see is what you will re-create." Work hard on adjusting real vision. The distortion of miasm repeats itself like a bad broken record, disrupting harmonies, corrupting the primal order of things, impeding the natural evolutionary process, blocking our soul growth, and overriding our conscious soul integration.

Karma and miasm can be viewed as chaotic, incoherent energetic patterns in our energetic fields. In contrast, divine right order represents a coherent energetic organization that reconnects us to our divine imprint. Miasm has blocked energy, which separates and impedes the free energetic flow from the source to *us*. The separation caused by miasms causes great suffering, such as diseases and sicknesses of body and mind.

Remedy

The use of homeopathy remedies is very effective in treating our physical ailments caused by miasms. However, it works best if we are not loaded or burdened with toxins and are implementing a good diet. There are four different diagnoses in homeopathy for this kind of miasmic therapy. A professional homeopathic doctor should be able to help you handle your complaints, effectively remove adverse effects from miasm, harmonize and bring balance to your emotion and mind, and even move the treatment beyond the body to enter the genetic programing at its root. Everything is energy. There is nothing else other than energy.

6

DETOXIFICATION AND DISCOVERING A HEALING SYSTEM WITHIN OUR BODY TEMPLATE

"You have to take seriously the notion that understanding the Universe is your responsibility because the only understanding of the Universe that will be useful to you is your own understanding."

— TERRENCE MCKENNA

This chapter will give you how things should unfold to start the journey of deep healing for yourself. The health steps are essential to clear your body of stagnant energy blocks properly. A cleaner and lighter body works better for energetic healing to be administered (life for homeopathy, bio-resonance) and will also take any form of healing to a higher level of success. I will show you different methods I have used for myself, my patients, and my family members.

DETOX YOUR BODY FIRST

Detoxification is a considerable part of your physical healing program. Heavy and toxic metals are enemies of your body, and they are everywhere: water, vaccines, food, old dental work, and the air we breathe. My patients are in their fifties, and some still have some lead amalgam left in their mouths. I ask them to have it removed by a particular dentist who knows how to perform this kind of work. You don't want to remove lead improperly – if done poorly; the toxins go back in your mouth and back into your bloodstream.

After we spotted the heavy metal problem, my fibromyalgia patients felt

45 to 50 percent better concerning their fatigue and pain in a short period, just by taking their detox seriously. There are many ways to do that – changing the food you eat to organic food (if possible) and purchasing a good detox supplement are examples. You can do these things at home, and they're not dangerous as long as you take the time to inform yourself and trust your inner guidance.

When treating my fibromyalgia patients, I found on my incredible Sensitiv Imago scan from Ukraine that the hypothalamus/pituitary glands and tissues were affected by a high amount of lead and mercury, mycoplasma toxins, and other heavy metals. Their entire bodies were also heavy metal loaded, which I suspect was why, due to toxins and lactic acid elimination, their muscles were so sore and painful after working out.

When our body is overloaded with all the heavy metals from smoking, car exhaust, dental amalgams, food, or water, it overloads our respiratory system and affects the nervous system as well. There is a strong reaction to it, of course, because our nervous system reacts strongly by sending signals throughout our body as fatigue or nerve pain. No, I'm not a medical doctor, but I can tell you that just by removing your heavy metals, you will not suffer as much after that. If you have fibromyalgia and you are a smoker, stop and detox. I use an herbal patch detox for my smoking patients and remove their lung toxins with bio-resonance tools. I even found heavy metals in the scans of nonsmokers as well.

In 2008, I was diagnosed with Hashimoto's disease, an autoimmune disease affecting the thyroid. According to current medical knowledge, there is *no* cure! Yikes! Most of my symptoms were similar to fibromyalgia: insomnia, weight loss, anxiety, depression, inability to concentrate (I could not meditate at all during that time), foggy brain, paranoia, unbalanced hormones, tachycardia, fatigue, and unexpected painful body cramps. On top of all that, I had a massive panic attack while driving in the middle of I-95. Those attacks happened three to four times a week.

Do these symptoms ring a bell to you? My nervous system was under attack from lead/mercury poisoning! I feared driving my car for a while because I never knew when my panic attacks would happen. My joy and happiness went out the window.

At first, I prescribed four different kinds of medicine: one for pain, one for the thyroid, one for the heart, and one for my anxiety. I tried to swallow those for two weeks, but they made me feel so sick that I ditched them (not quickly enough). After all the tests were performed, I got a gloomy prognosis from my endocrinologist. According to him, the solution was to surgically remove my thyroid, use radiation to destroy it, and be on medication for the rest of my life.

It was a significant turning point. My life as a healer began then. Learning to heal me then, was my prime purpose.

I went home, stopped taking my meds (please don't do this unless you talk to your doctor), and did my homework to understand where this went wrong in the first place. After all, I was fine before this problem occurred. Since I was a licensed acupuncturist, I had a better understanding of how health works (at least my own) and intuitively knew how toxins could seriously damage my health. I removed all of my previous amalgams from my mouth (use serious holistic dentistry if you do this). I detoxed my entire body of all the heavy metals I stored in the past due to my toxic behavior of smoking. I removed parasites, and I even flushed my liver and gall bladder three times. I worked hard to improve my diet; I juiced vegetables. I received acupuncture and Chinese herbs as treatments to balance my thyroid. In the process, I became more deeply involved in spiritual matters, and I had psychic work done twice on my throat chakra. Now, all these ordeals are history. I'm perfectly fine; I went from having Hashimoto's disease to having nothing in six months.

To detox most of my patients, we had recourse with chlorella, green drinks, wheatgrass, etc., and drinking lots of water. You can find pH strips online to measure your saliva's pH and see how much you should regulate it. Many methods and products are offered for detoxification to safely remove toxins, such as zeolite, charcoal, bentonite clay bath, parsley drops, cilantro drops, and high-PPM colloidal silver (atomic size), and homeopathy.

Important notice: do *not* take all of these at once. You don't want to go to a full detox too fast, especially if you do this for the first time. We performed detox through the skin as well with an infrared sauna. Any form of sweating is useful to alleviate the lymphatic system. Acupuncture and energetic work with the Rife machine, green drinks, liver cleanses, intestinal cleanses, colon cleanses, and a kidney cleanse will provide detoxification. All of them are utilized to clean the whole organ system.

Use lymphatic drainage and massage in-between to drain out toxins and drink a lot of water. Ask your doctor/ nurse practitioner/ medical spa about the various IV detox programs that are also effective at detoxing your liver and boosting your immune system.

All my patients are resilient now and are doing so many things on their own. They truly are detox veterans. We are in constant communication, and I keep a close watch on their progress. Their victories are my victories. All of us are plagued by heavy metals, and all your attempts to do proper detoxification will undoubtedly pay off. If you are not a health practitioner, I recommend having an alternative doctor follow your detoxification and healing progress and monitor you. And of course, don't do this alone at the beginning if you feel uncomfortable doing so.

LIVER AND GALL BLADDER FLUSH

The liver is a mighty organ. Please consider doing the liver cleanse as it is the largest solid organ and the largest gland in the human body. The liver helps in detoxification and is a part of the digestive system. The roles of the liver include protein synthesis and the production of chemicals. In Chinese medicine, the liver organ regulates and smooths the emotions when healthy. Alcohol consumption of any kind will deteriorate your liver rapidly.

This step to flush this organ is an important one – it will remove pain, raise and boost your immune system and improve your digestive system I used this methodology for years, for every patient and also for myself. If you have never done this, it is wise to do two (or three) flushes one month apart for the first year and at least once a year after that as maintenance. Pain such as heavy legs, sciatic pain, neck, back, and shoulder pain can be helped or eliminated with this detox. A clean and healthy liver will give you a sense of calmness and the ability to meet and assess stress with poise.

I never met a patient who knew about this simple cleanse. It eliminates so much of their pain. I can detect with my scans if my patients need it, but I know we all need to do it. If you eat fried potatoes or deep-fried food, such as chicken parmesan, chicken tenders, fried calamari, bread and butter, pancakes, etc., you need to do this.

It takes a little preparation, but the recipe is simple. When you decide to start the flush, purchase a "parasite cleanse" online that includes three ingredients: cloves, wormwood, and walnut hulls.

• On Days 1–3, take one capsule two times a day with meals.

• On Days 4–6, take two capsules two times a day with meals.

• On Days 7–10, take two capsules three times a day with meals.

• On Days 11–13, take three capsules three times a day with meals.

• On Day 14, take four capsules three times a day with meals. Do this step until you finish the bottle you purchased.

If you feel any discomfort, go back to a lower number of capsules, stay at a comfortable number for your body, and finish the bottle you have purchased.

Once you finish the whole bottle, stay home. Do not wait and start the following day with:

• Fresh organic grapefruit, (if you have a problem with grapefruit use lemon instead) Epsom salt, and olive oil. On that day, try not to eat anything too heavy at breakfast and lunch.

• Stop eating all together at 1:00 p.m.

• At 4:00 p.m., mix one and a half teaspoons of Epsom salt with eight ounces of water. Drink the mix.

• At 6:00 p.m., mix another one and a half teaspoons of Epsom salt with eight ounces of water. Drink the mix

• At 8:00 p.m., repeat the same mix of Epsom salt and water and drink it.
o You will be using the bathroom a lot, so it's a good idea to stay home.

• At 10:00 p.m., Juice and use 3/4 cup of organic grapefruit + 3/4 cup of (organic) olive oil, mix the combined ingredients together in a blender. Drink the mixture slowly (use a straw) within 15/20 minutes and get ready for bed. Try to go to sleep on your right side.

• It is important that you fall asleep fast, use natural melatonin or CBD if necessary. The liver works better by getting rid of the stones when we sleep.

• The following day, at 6:00 a.m., repeat the mixture. Mix one and a half teaspoons of Epsom salt with eight ounces of water. Drink the mix and wait for the flush.

• After the flush done, resume with breakfast

The stones will be flushed out after that. They are a mixture of bile and cholesterol clogging the liver and gall bladder duct, and they reduce their ability to cleanse and digest our food. It will be floating, and the colors could be black, brown, or green. I know people who, at fifty-five, had to have their gall bladder removed because they had a gall bladder crisis. It's not a good idea to have it removed. We need all our organs in their place and functioning. Resume eating after that reasonably.

PARASITE CLEANSE

Parasites are much more common than you think. We are all more or less affected by those foreign invaders. The CDC estimates hundreds of thousands of people have been infected in America, and many of us don't even know it. They come in a variety of forms and lodge themselves in our bodies, intestines, and organs. They feed on our blood, supplements, and vitamins and create all kinds of problems on the skin and during digestion. They can cause anything from fatigue to diarrhea.

In purchasing your parasite cleanse, you have to look for these three ingredients in the product: black walnut hulls, cloves, and wormwood. Look for something with the strength to kill and expel those parasites out of your body. You can contact them from a doorknob, contaminated water, undercooked meat (especially pork, known to host more bacteria), and contaminated fruits. Parasites create havoc on our health and immune system.

I recommend doing a parasite cleanse four times a year, just like the seasons. Keep doing it, too. You eat all the time, and the chances you are getting parasites are pretty high unless you're a health freak. Even though I treated back pain and neck pain just by removing parasites with a homeopathic remedy and acupuncture treatment, they don't require much detoxing if the patient is pretty healthy already.

What are the signs of removing parasites? Feeling bloated after food intake, bad breath, toenail fungus, smelly feet, and skin problems are some of the signs and symptoms; just be watchful of your skin, as skin is the body's biggest organ, and a good indicator of parasitic infection.

According to Dr. Hulda Clark, in her book *The Cure for All Diseases*, "All disease is caused by foreign organisms and pollutants that damage the immune system." She mentioned that eliminating these organisms from the body using herbal supplements or electrical means while removing pollutants from the diet would cure most of our symptoms."

Parasites have a consciousness and are attracted to what is capable of attracting them. They thrive in their host because they can. Maintaining hygiene when cooking food is highly recommended to maintain healthy guts and organs. We have to continually monitor the number of parasites, fungus, candida, yeast, and mold in our body to maintain good gut habits.

Let's be clear about this: one size medicine does not fit all. Find your precise need with your doctor to find out if you have parasites, viruses, fungi, bacteria, yeast, candida, or heavy metals. Remove them safely. Do not do guesswork on your own.

NUTRITION – FOOD IS IMPORTANT, QUANTITY IS MORE IMPORTANT

Let's tackle nutrition. It concerns most of our life, and our survival depends on it. Growing up in France – one of the richest places for culinary arts in the world – I was one of a few accidentally "lucky" children. I grew up in an area where money was not abundant. I mean by "lucky" that I could not experience all the food I wanted to eat growing up, including sugar, meat, cream, cheese, and desserts; nor could I have rich, fatty food or palatable food. Therefore, I never developed a taste for tasty, rich, or sugary food.

The menu available to me was always simple. I grew up having the same food Monday to Sunday, and it was repeated for seven to eight years after that until I was moved to another French province. In my teenage years, for about three years on and off, I often went hungry weeks at a time as I grew up by myself at the age of sixteen. I asked my classmates for any food they could spare, and I ate whatever was available at that time. Sometimes, I only ate one time each day; sometimes, I ate nothing.

I naturally and involuntarily learned to conserve energy as I survived those years with just bread and zucchini. I learned to adapt to the situation by accepting the idea that it's okay if my body is not receiving food right then. I developed strength and a deep appreciation for food when I had it. Did I lack nutrition? Oh, certainly. But I caught up on the nutrition deprivation later on as an adult, minus the super taste buds I could have built but did not. This "sad" part of my life turned out to be a real savior.

I'm not going to tell you what exactly you need to eat. You can find a nutritionist for that if you choose to and get a diet tailored to your blood type. I can say that you should stay away from all foods that are not organic or not derived from nature. Eliminate canned food – it has toxic preservatives. Go for fiber and reach for leafy vegetables and organic fruits. Build a simple, tasty menu and teach yourself to appreciate simple food. Eat slow, be present with your food, and eat with deep, conscious awareness. It took lots of people to grow your food and lots of solar sun energy, which is now entering your energetic system.

If you have intense cravings for your "killer" food, find a good substitute for it. The desire will go away as you implement meditation and focus your mind on something else. Eat small quantities throughout the day and stop eating at 6:00 p.m. The body repairs best at night when allowed to do so. If you go to bed feeling full, your body won't have much time and energy to repair itself. Because your digestive system is slow, you wake up feeling tired. If your digestion is impaired, take some good digestive enzymes with your meals, especially if your meal consists of carbs and meat.

As adults who supposedly acquired knowledge, how can we not see that we live in a sick, food-addicted world? Forget about the people who are addicted to cigarettes – we focus on them like they alone have an addiction. Lots of us have strong addictions to sugar, alcohol, deep-fried food, or other potent stimulants, just to name a few.

Slow down on caffeine – choose decaf or herbal tea, or eliminate it. Get rid of sugary sodas and anything that mentions "diet" on the label. The sugar substitute in many diet products will, in time, affect your thinking. Matcha green tea is an excellent substitute for coffee.

Food is a discipline and should be carefully monitored. Unhealthy food also affects your meditation and even clogs your physical energetic pathways big time. Your attainment to reach your greater Self will be long and hard, if not impossible. Watch for anything that will bring defects to your mind, such as bad news, media, too much TV, fluorite in toothpaste, negative thoughts, negative beliefs, FEAR, and so on.

Our supermarkets have more food than we can think of, and we keep creating more food substitutes to outsmart ourselves. We believe dieting will make us healthier. Diet this, diet that, low calorie this, low calorie that – we keep eating for taste because our life is not that yummy. We eat to stuff our stomachs so we don't feel the emptiness created by deep, unresolved psychological cravings. We know about all the disastrous statistics of our health nationwide: childhood obesity, diabetes, tasteless food grown in polluted environments. When I go into a supermarket, I realize there are only one or two things energetically viable and useful: organic fresh vegetables and fruits, nuts, and grains.

Just eat one group of food at a time. Different food needs different digestive enzymes. Eat your fruit/desserts alone and eat your protein/ salads together, but don't include potatoes and rice, for example. Rice, beans, and meat? Bad combo. Sweet plantains, cheese, potatoes, and meat? Also, bad.

In my ongoing experience, milk, meat, or products with hormones that increase quantity and durability rather than quality and are overabundant in supermarkets create an imbalance within the endocrine system. It is not uncommon to see young adults having blocked lymph nodes with a hormonal system on overdrive. The list of health problems caused by our food system is overwhelming.

Overeating is a disease in the West. We are hungry all the time. We are hungry for everything. We don't know what, in truth, we are truly hungry for. We are living our lives so unaware of the real hunger within. We are on autopilot, guided by ads, media, cravings, and habits.

We grew up guided only by automatic, unconscious parents and societies and became frustrated adults later in life. We use food as a substitute for growth. It is easier to stuff ourselves all day long with things we like, rather than looking for change. The food we have been eating for so long has already altered our minds and left us with no substantial growth desire.

Could it be that we need to taste more *love* in our life instead? The more we eat, the sleepier we get. This is because the body needs a tremendous amount of energy to digest all that we ate. If what we ate was pizza and a Coke, the body goes into a "coma" state because digestion is hard to cope with.

In Ayurvedic philosophy, there are three different food awareness states: tamas, which means dense darkness; rajas, which means destruction/chaos; and sattva, which means goodness/balance. This could be to overlay on our lifestyle, mind/personality, choices, and so on. The category we need to achieve to balance and heal in should be of the sattvic quality. The world is oscillating between tamas and Rajas, and we need to gain more of the pure sattvic state.

At the time of writing this book, I have ten-year-old twins. Like lots of kids, my kids love candy and pizza (which were introduced at school, thanks to the system in place!), and they don't always listen to my advice, but I know they will listen to their schoolteacher. I went to her to discuss how to get children to eat better in their class. It takes a whole village to raise our kids; they can learn from more than one source. Like playing billiards, sometimes you have to find an indirect course to hit the ball and reach your target.

In Japan, mealtime is a big deal at school. Teachers educate children in healthy meals at a young age – we agree that the younger they learn, the better. All children in Japan are responsible for participating in cooking their lunch. They all know about sharing, delegating, cleaning, and tidying up after themselves. Their school lunch menu consists of delicious vegetable soups, soba noodles, tofu, sea vegetable broths, etc. The oldest living person there is a 117-year-old Japanese lady.

The whole message here is food should be deliciously light and simple. If you learn to live by this method, it will save you money and you will stay healthier because your immune system can thrive on simple, digestible things. Even going to bed a little hungry is best. Fast once a week if you can, as our Bible suggests. It's healthy!

Simple foods, I think, are best for us. The simpler, the better. If you are accustomed to certain types of food that make you sick and you know it, stop eating them. If you like potent stimulants like coffee, slow down your consumption – your nervous system will be on the red alert all day long, year after year. Substitute it for something milder, like bio coffee or green tea and honey.

Changing your food habits will not happen overnight, especially if it comes from a hard-to-kick, profound cultural aspect. Know also that if you have a big family, everyone is different. Some or all of your family members might be resistant to change. You can start by talking about it and bringing new information to them as you inform yourself. Be flexible and tolerant; don't become a drill sergeant all of a sudden because you think you are on to something great and, therefore, everybody should be on it too. Change yourself first and leave the others to God.

Most of us are going for the taste in food; the tongue is an organ devoid of wisdom, so we must train the mind. Meditation is the mediator between our senses and our greater Self. We will discuss meditation and why it is one of the most important remedies for our ills later.

Work on being aware of your food habits one day at a time. Your need for food intake is always different from someone else's. Use your intelligence to determine what it is that your body needs. If you experience chronic constipation, there could be something else more to eat, than eating bread and potatoes, as this will worsen the problem.

Change your food habit all by yourself. It's better if done silently. Suppose someone wants to follow your example, great! If not, that's fine too. It's not our job to change them (but you can write a book about it). I met so many people dishing on other people's food habits because they think theirs is better. We are not in a competition with anyone. The real *work* should happen silently within us – that is strength. You don't want to be an annoyance to anyone, and you respect all choices.

SPIRITUAL REMEDIES

We all live within the confines of our understanding of what life is based on from our upbringing, personal intelligence given at birth, and education. It seems that some people get more, some less, and some get none at all! In reality, the opportunity is the same for all. From my knowledge and experience as a healer, the consciousness of sickness or disease perceived by an individual at the level of their understanding of who they are playing an essential part in how and if they will heal. Is he/she the problem, or is he/she going to obliterate the problem by realizing that the supreme healer is himself/herself?

TAKE CARE OF THE MIGHTY MIND

Is the mind our best friend or worse enemy? Many masters teach about the mind and how to access it for good use instead of the other way around. We are led by our mind and our thoughts constantly, and they take us around and around uncontrollably, like a chimpanzee jumping from branch to branch, never stopping.

First, we need to understand how the mind works and how to stop it or slow it down. How do we reason with a cluttered mind? How do we work with a fixed mind? The mind is almighty, but for now, we are not using it to our advantage. A clear mind can go a long way.

Often, we worry, think about the future, and focus on what is not working in our life. A negative mind always goes to where something is not working, where something negative and worrisome is. It sees danger where there is none. It's cunning and deceiving. Its job is to protect the personality and keep us safe, but it can also destroy us.

When our mind is too much, it can become troublesome. Therefore, we need to teach our mind to be relaxed and obedient for our own good. You'll notice that when we fixate our mind on something insignificant long enough, it becomes magnified. A small thing can become enormous, and paranoia sets in if you let it run wild.

According to yogic thoughts, there are five stages to achieve mind control. The first stage is a distracted, scattered, and fragmented mind. The second stage is dull and forgetful. The third stage is the gathering state, which is occasionally steady and sometimes distracted. The fourth is a one-pointed mind state focusing only on one thing. The last step is the ability to control the mindfully.

The most significant impediment to concentration is giving in to restlessness and becoming scattered. To achieve a one-pointed mind, you have to train the mind to concentrate on one thing at a time and fully stay with it. It is primordial to introspect and observe the mind. When thoughts arise, watch them come and go. Do not wrestle with them – struggles will create more mental waves in the process. Persevere in the task. We discipline our minds with constant practice. You will gradually organize your mind and extend the concentration and move into meditation.

When I undertook meditation, I would stare at a candle flame to keep my mind from wandering. Of course, it was going left and right, but I just brought it back into focus and trained myself not to judge it. I started with fifteen minutes and slowly increased the time to thirty minutes, then one hour. It was a struggle to sit down and meditate for years.

Later, I found that digging for negative emotions and healing traumas helped me enter meditation quickly. My inner "baggage" was removed, and there was more space within myself. My mind was free to enter into calmness and set into meditation rapidly. There was more space, and it was way more enjoyable to meditate.

Besides the focus and achieving one-pointedness, meditation is the best way to rest the entire nervous system. We disconnect from the world by going within and withdrawing our five senses. All our body systems get deep rest and can perform better afterward. It is a misconstrued idea that meditation is doing nothing even though it can appear this way.

When we go within through the meditation process, lots of movements are happening at the same time within ourselves, yet we feel the perfect stillness. But it takes practice to recognize that. It is action in inaction. Our whole life within and without is being reorganized at the same time. It is a reset button for change. When all is calm and peaceful within, the outside world will mirror that back to us. Don't take my word for it. Try it – you won't regret it. But give it some time to take root. Do the work to reach the Self that is beyond the mind.

I had a friend who was a lovely person; she felt she smoked too much and desired to quit but never succeeded at it, no matter how many times she tried. After enrolling with a group of Buddhist meditators, I was so delighted that she naturally kicked the habit without a patch after a year of starting meditation.

When I saw her again, her face was glowing, her skin looked radiant, and

I could see the dark, murky aura caused by her heavy smoking in the past was no more to be seen or felt. Group energy is a powerful supporter in your endeavor to grow if you don't like to do things alone. A group is influential in helping you activate the practice and will carry you if you feel discouraged. Keeping the company of high levels of frequency and conscious people is always preferred to share common ground and grow. Indeed, one candle can light another.

MEDITATION

To meditate is to let go of the world and the mind to merge into the Infinite. It can be done at any time that seems fit. Sitting up with the spine erect is necessary. Keeping the mind awake and alert without falling asleep is the goal here. Meditation is better early in the morning because the atmosphere is more conducive to peace and quietness, but if you cannot do it in the morning, choose an appropriate time.

If done every day at the same time and place, you will build a tremendous ability to go into silence rapidly. The mind will just slip into meditation immediately. I do mine every night after my kids go to bed. I let go of everything from the day and dive into relaxing the mind by breathing and concentrating on the third eye.

If stopping the mind is difficult for you at first, below is a useful exercise I learned from Guru Ma in New Delhi to block all thoughts from coming and going, which keeps your mind busy to the point of making yourself sick. This technique will help you experience within yourself the silence between two thoughts. This is called the silent gap.

Exercise to Stop Thoughts

Sit in a comfortable chair or on your bed with your legs crossed and your arms at your side. Keep your back straight and relax your neck, shoulders, and entire body. Center yourself in your third eye at the pituitary center. If you feel your mind acting up, you can mentally tell yourself just to relax. Breathe slowly and calmly. Empty the mind.

Your thoughts might flare up even more during this exercise. Just watch your thoughts come and go. Don't judge; let them be. Just be in the moment with your breath. Something is watching those thoughts come and go; *this* is what we will try to feel more in time by expanding the gap between two thoughts.

Now, slowly take a deep, controlled breath through your nose. When you cannot inhale anymore, hold your breath as long as you possibly can. While holding your breath, just use your ears to *listen* to any kind of noise around you. Listening during this exercise is essential. It will make you more present and aware.

Then slowly exhale. Repeat this for at least fifteen minutes and expand the time to thirty minutes. It will teach you to stop the mind from being so active; therefore, the meditation will be easier to perform after this exercise.

When you don't breathe and hold your breath, thoughts automatically stop. But you need to be aware of the sounds around you. The act of listening intensely will help you increase your awareness exponentially. When you do this exercise, the mind stops, and it will be just a short time that you can sense or feel the real *you* – the Presence.

Now, after the thought-blocking exercise, you can enter into meditation. Just quietly breathe and listen to your breath going in and out. Focus on your third eye in the middle of your forehead and fix your mind here. Let go and let God.

Do not analyze anything; become blank. It feels good not to have control of anything. Become, in your heart, a little child for its divine parent. In time, with silence, you will build more of a relationship with your Inner Being/God. It will slowly speak to you and awaken you to be able to see from within.

Any healing and transformation you achieve will be validated with meditation practice. The experience of stillness is not one to be sought after; instead, let it come naturally to you. Let go of all expectations here. There is nothing else you want other than *being* one with *it*.

I started meditation at the age of twenty-six. At that time, I was consuming coffee, meat, and cigarettes, and my thinking mind was always hectic, like an ongoing roller coaster. When I closed my eyes, I could feel my mind racing and go in many different directions at once nonstop. It took me such a long time to calm it down before I could enter into meditation. To slow the mind down, we need to give up certain foods. That will assist us with meditation because consuming the right food is important to meditation. There are no adverse side effects to practicing meditation. All your electric wiring will work better, and meditation is the enabler for your mind to heal. By gathering thoughts and allowing your mind to reorganize itself, you will heal your body. When the mind heals, the body does too.

The self-effort engineered by staying still creates waves of peace that, in turn, boomerang back to you and your life. The hectic energy that occupies your busy mind will gradually settle, just like a peaceful lake. People are surprised when "bad" things happen to them. It is the creative mind sending them back their creation in constant unconscious motion. Watch the thought and the mind; we emit as vibration, which then comes back to us. If there is one crucial thing about meditation to know, meditation is the glue that binds all of your practice to get better or heal and make everything a success. I combine silent meditation with mantras and chakra meditation as well. This triple combo is a bomb to send you like a rocket ship into the God zone. Hands up!

When I was revisiting the country I was born in, I observed a holy man walking with slow movements in the middle of the busiest street in Ho Chi Minh (previously called Saigon). He went on and on for hours, days, and weeks. Every time I went to that section of the town, he was there, walking the whole street in slow motion. It took him the entire day to walk the entire street. Each movement was like a man walking on the moon. Later on, I understood its significance; I'm sure he was making a statement about ripples.

It was a conscious meditation in movement. The slow part shows that the less movement we create in our daily life, the fewer ripples come back to us. We also can learn to live our life aware of each of our movements, awake and present in a meditation of perpetual motion. Slow down in what we do, simplify our lives, enjoy more of everything, and rest in silence. A journey of a thousand steps starts with just one. We can start by being absolutely present with only ten slow steps as a moving meditation that can increase to more steps later on as you become more still within.

FUTURISTIC MEDITATION

I wanted to share this information with my reader about meditation using the 2021 meditation version offered nowadays, with virtual reality (VR). You can smile about this, but I know how difficult it is for most beginners to stay still and meditate; therefore, I find this tool an easy solution for those who need more visuals and sounds and can be done with VR. I have set my kids to do meditation with this technique, and besides the fact that they love it, I get them to be cool kids now, and it works best for them. We can be firm in teaching meditation and use flexibility in our ways to get there. Today technologies help us with many things to be accomplished in extraordinary ways. I know that in our future, we can look at VR as a means to disengage from a noisy world and quickly connect with ourselves; this allows us to reach different parts of our brains to heal and connect with our Universe within and deeply relax. So, if you already own the Oculus 2, just purchase the app Tripp or Flow, and it will teach you a fantastic way to go zen in no time. It is still better not to become addicted to VR (games), but if this can provide you thirty minutes or more of deep mind rest and connection within your Self, then go for it.

THE SEVEN ENERGETIC CENTERS (CHAKRAS) AND KUNDALINI

Kundalini is the cosmic power in individual bodies. It is not electricity or magnetism; it is a culmination of life force activated in meditative experiences by performing all yoga forms. It is better suited to practice kundalini under the grace of a guru or an experienced teacher but alone is alright too, as long as you use precise learning tools available out there.

Kundalini can be activated and rise through the spine through a psychic channel called *Sushumna Nadi* (located in the spinal cord). Its structure is greatly purified. It is a spiritual potential of raw cosmic power and cannot be taken lightly. Premature attempts to awaken this dormant energy can be dangerous if you are not prepared for it.

I experienced a slow and steady awakening of the kundalini. Even though I was incredibly prepared and worked through it, I remember when that power rose within me at 2:00 a.m. I felt a little panicky and did not feel I could handle it all at once all by myself. I quickly got up and moved around to shake it off. At the time, the spiritual kundalini was so strong and powerful, and I thought my mind would completely lose it if I were not prepared to breathe, relax, and let myself go through the experience.

The awakening of kundalini typically happens gradually, moving up slowly from one chakra to another one. The energy can be raised to the third eye but does not stay there for a long time unless you are a pure yogi. Lots of effort and concentration has to happen before it can take place.

From the third eye to the top of the head, kundalini's last step is God's total divine union. But it doesn't stay long either; we need to keep practicing and become purified and adept at keeping it there. It is the last step of complete liberation.

Throughout your body are six main energy wheels we call chakras, starting from your tail bone and going up to the seventh one, which is stationed at the top of your head. Each center has served a growth purpose since the day we are born, and with due practice, we keep growing spiritually to reach the top of our head as the sublime experience and union with our divine Self (God). They are connected by a fine energetic cord (*Sushumna*), which lets unimpeded energy, when ready, flow from the first chakra to the seventh chakra and lead the person to perfect union with the divine Self. At the base of the sacral bone, there is a dormant energy called kundalini that, when awakened, ascends and energizes each of the seven centers, propelling a person into this divine union.

There are color and sound vibrations within each chakra as well. But using the spiritual sound "om" for each energy vortex while doing the meditation, mentally or out loud, will activate the corresponding chakra and keep your mind moving to each one.

I firmly believe that the ideal normal evolution of man starts from childhood (me, myself, and I – first chakra), moving to adulthood (second, third, and fourth), and then Godhood (fifth, sixth, and seventh). We all know that most of us end up dying old and sick; therefore, the step toward enlightenment is significantly slowed down. Hence reincarnation.

There is an appointed time for everyone's energetic center (EC) to be activated, functioning, opened, and balanced for us to move their life forward and experience a full and godly existence. In my humble belief and observation, that hot flash is the kundalini energy attempt to rise through the spine, but we are not prepared for it at all. The blocks within our entire body system are not energetically and spiritually prepared for its ascent. Therefore, the cleansing/ purifying work of the kundalini rising through a body is cluttered by toxins creating what we call "menopausal symptoms."

We were not meant to physically age that fast; because of our connection to it, a human can be compared to nature; let's just observe a 150-year-old tree. It continues still to bear leaves; year after year, the trunk gets more substantial and thicker. But with humans, the ability to reproduce healthy cells year after year is lost after about twenty years; to live past 100 years becomes impossible for most. Our morphogenetic energy template is not working and has been in a state of defect for a long time. Our DNA is working in reverse instead of rewinding itself as it should.

The collective human understanding of how we age forces us all into a deep hypnotic state, to a place we think we cannot escape, such as aging and sickness. Can't we question everything and form our thought patterns and beliefs that are truer to us and remove those false beliefs that keep us so small? Our intelligence should not be limited by the teaching received from beings who were oblivious to the untold *truth*.

Now, with so much spiritual energy and knowledge happening in the world to assist us, in this massive awakening, is the time when we can still reconnect all of our wirings and plug into a live system beyond our little understanding (for now) and rise above human limitation.

I recommend working with the chakras. Those innate body systems can bring great power to access and awaken the dormant Self and bless us with a life of attainments beyond our dreams, independent of worldly possession and attachments of any kind. When awakened, a Self is sufficient to itself with its perfect balance.

I received initiation myself, and practicing it for five years led my little Self to experience the extent of this raw power within us all. There is a world of silence and wonder to be discovered beyond what any words can express. The Presence is real and accessible to anyone seeking *it*. Experiencing the Self forces the deepening of an understanding that cannot be revealed or talked about even if I try to explain. As soon as it is expressed through words, its inaccessible deep feeling is lost. It becomes somehow empty. It is a full godly experience to behold. When we reach this state, there is no need for words.

The definition of each chakra and what it provides us with to support our life growth is astonishing. Each chakra works in helping our entire existence from work to love of God. It provides us with the supreme power behind every step we need to arrive at our destination. We want those chakras to work correctly to experience power and guidance within our system.

There's a lot to say about chakras, but I just give a brief description and gentle guidance in this book. It's best to experience them by yourself through meditation. Experience is knowledge, and knowledge is power. As we mature and grow spiritually, everything within our higher Self will be revealed for us to understand and divinely know. Reading someone else's experience is not yours to own.

According to known masters in the East, there are 114 major chakras in the body. Two are outside the physical body. Those 112 chakras take us across a world to another; 108 chakras can be worked with, and four are not needed. They are doorways to divine knowledge. The more chakras we have fully operating, the more we enter our super nature, even developing superpowers like Jesus. Only 21 chakras are needed to operate the body, but most people know only seven main chakras, and we don't even fully utilize all of those.

TAKING A LOOK AT THE SEVEN MAIN CHAKRAS

First Chakra – Muladhara

Located in the sacral plexus, this chakra, when balanced, can support our survival, our sense of knowing, and our feeling of security and direction in life. It unlocks mind control, knowledge of more profound truth, and the like. When a child is devoid of love and basic needs from parental guidance or goes through violence, this chakra will be wounded, which, in addition to lots of other problems, means his/her development will be reduced or completely stuck. He/she will have difficulty providing for himself/herself later in life.

Second Chakra – Swadhisthana

Located in the genital area, this chakra affects relationships, sexuality, love for the Self, confidence, power, intuition, and psychic knowledge. I have witnessed many women who have problems within the second center because of psychic attachment or attachment to an abusive relationship. Anything that reduces a person's power, like being controlled by your parents of an abusive husband/ or relationship that overpower you, will wound and disrupt this energy center. It creates uterine problems for women, causing this center to leak energy and become significantly weakened.

Women come from a long history of being dominated by men physically and mentally, nullifying their ability to get in touch with their inner divine feminine and power. Processing this center to full awakening and removing all destructive blocks can bring women to know their Self profoundly and live a life of interdependence without being needy. It will provide inner strength and direction and will allow them to understand their potential as an individual.

If this chakra is not working correctly, the adverse side effects are aggressiveness and powerlessness. The power needed to move ahead in life and grow will be hindered, and in terms of birthing a new Self, life will come to a stop.

Third Chakra – Manipura

Located at the navel, this chakra controls the health of the entire body. It is a powerful center to activate because it is a spiritual brain that can regulate our emotions and stress. Total control of this chakra bestows perfect health on the practitioner. This chakra is not working well if you experience stomach and digestion problems, which I have seen in many instances working with my patients. Healing will happen if this energetic center is working correctly at all times.

Fourth Chakra – Anahata

Located at the heart center, this chakra reigns over love, compassion, complete understanding, and divine and unconditional love experiences. I do not mean by this the conditional human love we all experience. I mean the pure, unselfish cosmic love for all creation.

It is essential to activate this heart center because it is the bridge of our Earthly connection with the divine connection throughout the body in lower and higher chakras. Nothing works well or fully functions if this center is not fully open and activated.

Fifth Chakra – Vishuddhi

Located at the base of the throat, this center will help manifest desires in healthy communication, completing projects, and creativity when properly aligned with the second chakra. You can speak with in-depth knowledge about the Self. It gives us the ability to express our highest truths with kindness and without holding back. It knows who we are at all times.

I used to have problems with this center and developed Hashimoto's disease. After I aligned myself with physical and spiritual healing, my life moved forward, more aligned and centered in my truth, and I gained the ability to express myself more freely. Chakras are an ongoing system that needs to be sustained every day of our lives because we have not reached full enlightenment yet. The energy can partially come up to the third eye but will not remain there until we reach the perfect divine Union's final stage with the Self. It is daily cultivation.

Sixth Chakra – Ajana

This chakra is located between the eyebrows. A spiritual teacher told me, "He who meditates successfully on this center destroys the karma of all past lives and becomes a liberated soul." We develop intuition and psychic powers when we just concentrate in this center and chant "Om." The frontal lobe is home to the sixth chakra; it is the epicenter of Knowing (with a capital K) within the yoga/ chakra system. We need to consciously relax this frontal lobe to get all the benefits from meditation. Damage in this region will result in significant challenges for our mental health.

Seventh Chakra – Sahasrara

This chakra is at the top of the head. I always thought of this chakra as the best way to exit the body. We can escape from this chakra if we meditate well and we are connected with our soul. We can go at the time of our physical death and exit through this chakra. It will be a conscious death. It is a chakra of extreme bliss that creates a mindful state and the place of the highest knowledge.

All chakras, of course, have their importance and reason to be. They are divine cosmic helpers in terms of life force and intelligence. They are all connected and interconnected; they all need to be activated and working for us to witness their ability to propel us into a godly life. All is in place within our body to use with intelligence and wisdom. The chakra system is a mighty one to be acquainted with.

There are many paths to lead us to the supreme truth. If there is only one thing I practice every day (besides eating sensibly), it is the chakra system. The invisible force behind it sets everything into motion; it helps us accomplish specific tasks easier and even provides the serious seeker with the necessity.

I started on the path of kundalini yoga in 2000, learned the science behind it (just like I do for everything else in life), and moved on to a more complex chakra meditation, which provided me with remarkable growth within two years. Once those chakras are working the right way, and we are receptive to their energy, we can harness that energy to manifest anything we need in our life or grow as fast as we should. They have a force of attraction of their own; there is nothing to force. Everything becomes easy and automatic. Growth can happen quickly. This has been my experience.

SHAKTIPAT IS A SOUL REMEDY: LIFE FORCE TRANSMISSION

In the world of mystics, adding more rich spiritual experiences, if we can, is a great thing. *Shaktipat* is an energy to be received and felt by transmission from a perfected master to a true seeker wanting to awaken his/ her kundalini. These masters still exist, but few are truly genuine, so discrimination is called for if you choose to embark on this journey of kundalini awakening.

Kundalini energy holds so many powerful blessings that can fully awaken you in a shorter time. Let's be clear here: we are not living in a "perfect" world that allows us to free our schedule and perform the highest form of work within six years or less. Unless you are born as an Avatar, fully awakened and immune to the law of karma, there is a lot of work ahead.

If someone dedicated himself/herself to shadow work already and weeded out all negativity and purified his/ her mind and heart, *Shaktipat* will offer tremendous and quick help. Otherwise, the process will take much longer. It depends on how open and where you are spirituality wise. Kundalini frees our being by perfecting our body template, filling the mortal frame with pure life force, and taking you from mortal man to immortal conscious being. It's priceless.

In the past, when there was no internet or COVID-19, I was willing to fly all around the world to find answers to this deep inner quest. Every attempt in my spiritual pursuit led me to understand that our thirst for real knowledge will always be provided with divine help along the way that meets our every need, whether it is money or serendipitous meetings with the right master. Spend that money to learn and grow; don't be a miser on the path to find God. Being too thrifty (based on fear of lack) will undermine our spiritual progress as we acknowledge lack instead of universal abundance providing for our every need. We can just open up and trust the process. I know perfect faith is the only mighty missing ingredient for us to attract what we need in our lives quickly. Ye people of little faith, why are you so afraid?" said Jesus.

Trust your inner guidance and the perfect design of your existence. We are all universal children coming back "home" to our awaiting Father.

If this work takes us ten years or more, so be it if it's less than that, great! But let's forsake the expectation of a time frame or an outcome. We can miss what's important. It took one whole lifetime to move one or two main negative traits of a person on the path to perfection in ancient times. Today, we have the possibility to do it in one, providing a focused desire to attain.

If you still wonder about a time frame, some masters I know and read about abroad achieved this within six to seven years of a life cycle. But their spiritual training was gruesome. Honestly, I don't think we are cut out for that style of reaching enlightenment, as it demands lots of mind control. But we can do it with our style. The sky is the limit. Let's be creative. No matter what way you choose to do so, the moment you embrace this journey earnestly and wholeheartedly, your divine meeting will happen. At our level of conscious lifestyle and mindset, the more help we get from genuine spiritual masters, the better.

I started my self-discovery journey at twenty-six while living in Paris and experiencing two years of deep depression. I never saw then that Paris was one of the most beautiful places in the world; my mind was always in utter turmoil.

As I was walking one day in Rue des Ecoles, I stumble on an outside stall with books for sale. Thank God I love to read! Two books caught my eyes. One was about hatha yoga and one about Swami Vivekananda's teaching. Flipping through the pages, my eyes caught a few sentences; from there, everything within my spirit ignited. I went home with the book and read all through the night, eager to end this depression of mine.

My insomnia then turned to pure divine focus. I devoured those books like a starved child who had not eaten for years and felt like I discovered a remedy that, once upon a time, I knew existed. This was perfectly safe to do every day with only one sure side effect: liberation from suffering.

After the first week of my daily yoga and meditation routine from those books, I noticed calm and better breathing. But best of all was a pure and relaxed mind I thought I would never have. The depression was no more. I was able to reconnect myself daily to Source with its immense support in improving my health and mind. Since that serendipitous event thirty-two years ago, the little spark has been ignited to consume this ignorant little Self entirely. Like in an alchemical process, I willingly went through the journey to bring the most extraordinary transformation to myself, with an irreversible effect.

AYAHUASCA (DMT – DIMETHYLTRYPTAMINE)

I found this to be the quickest healing method I introduced to lots of people. I feel that ayahuasca's spirit molecules are another form of God in action.

DMT is a brew consumed with a shaman in the Amazon forest or, if you can find one, in your town (nothing is impossible). It is considered an illegal substance in the United States, but there is a Church of Ayahuasca in Orlando, Florida. DMT is a fascinating molecule that is studied and scientifically researched around the world. This powerful God's remedy provided by Mother Nature herself is known to help people with so many ailments, such as depression, anxiety, cancer, diabetes, and more.

If you don't want to spend time doing lots of searching and digging into what went wrong within your psyche in the past, an ayahuasca ceremony can provide lots of answers in one night. The catch is that you have to stay awake all night and work through puking or taking many trips to the bathroom (though that's not necessarily true for everyone).

I have experienced it many times (and still do). To my knowledge, it might help heal lots of fibromyalgia symptoms, as most of our health problems are created in our minds or are a result of long-term, unresolved hurt of the past. It will speed up your ascension toward the light. One night with ayahuasca removes ten years of your untold problems.

If you don't know what kind of problems you need to work on, don't worry. It does all the work for you: digging, healing, and procuring the exhilarating feeling of being one with everything, such as nature, animals, people, and so on when it's over. Keep in mind; everyone experiences things differently.

To me, this was the finding of a lifetime. My life in 2014 was seriously stuck and at a halt. I fell on my knees and pressed the Universe to show me a sure lead to end this paralyzing life where I felt no remarkable growth was happening. I did all the prayers, learnings, diggings, and work and went to all sorts of different therapies. Despite all this, I could not figure out the heck I was feeling or why I felt so alone. I was missing something big. I felt my life was caught in a maze once again, unable to bring myself up to the next step. My life was in limbo; it was like going to the grind every day and making it bearable enough that I could "survive" everything: love, work, kids, and all. I was not happy with myself at all!

I got angry with God that night, and I yelled at Him: "Why this? Why that? Why? Why? Why?" The messenger came to me rapidly one day after. A person I just met told me about ayahuasca, also called a "plant teacher," from the Amazon. A shaman was in the area to perform a ceremony. After listening to, whom I will call the "messenger," "I made all the arrangements to experience the plant within thirty minutes with few questions. I trusted the hunch, and it saved my life. Since then, nothing has been the same – for the better.

DMT is the spirit molecule that was theorized to be released by the pineal gland in small quantities naturally, so we all possess a small amount in our body. On the spiritual side, it facilitates the soul's journey to move in and out of the body. It is a complete surrender of the human mind to bring deep healing and exert a profound change in its behavior.

DMT is a powerful psychedelic, not to be taken lightly as it is a sacred medicine. It procures a near-death mystical experience. Many people witnessed profound mystical experiences; some became geniuses in their art and creativity afterward. Sometimes, others became more present and compassionate. Some even met with extraterrestrials and ascended masters!

Not me. My first seven to ten experiences with the spirit molecules were tough and hard. I felt compelled to endure journeys that were deeper than deep. All my spiritual windows were kicked wide open, and I experienced what I thought were the most challenging teachings of my life – but at the same time the most rewarding. I was eager for change, ready to release fear and conditioned existence. I was prepared for it all, and it taught me hard. I wanted out of this reality, either dead or alive. I was ready to take a considerable step now and leave this false identity behind at all costs. And nothing was going to stop me. I wanted more out of life; I wanted it all. I needed a step up in life with a different consciousness or an exit. This time, my life had become so unbearable and insipid, and I was feeling it. Ayahuasca will help you release all forms of control that are not helpful and experience life more from the heart center.

One particular time I experienced ayahuasca in 2017 on my birthday, a true third eye-opening. I was able to see (with my open eyes) the invisible yet light energy flowing from all the leaves, branches, and roots. It was a rare view of energy passing through every nook and crevasse of stone and grass. I felt like I was in the *Avatar* movie or my kid's video games. I saw the enchanted forest!

I was seeing a light show cascading along with trees and with branches and throughout nature. My window of altered perception showed me how much we don't see anything in its truest form. We cannot see our body of light because of our three-dimensional, dense perception, but that does not mean it's not there.

It was the first time I had such an incredible experience with ayahuasca, and it was most of the time difficult. I guessed *it* knew it was my birthday and, bestowed on me the gift. Drinking *yahe* (ayahuasca) took me by the hand and made me go through the Dark Night of the Soul. I felt like I died each time just to live again more fully the following day.

All that was necessary for me to see was revealed to me in clear, successive images, like a movie projected on my mind screen. I saw my entire past, childhood, teenage years, my present, and all the untold struggles I went through in life. It was so unbelievable! The spirit herb's intelligence knew precisely where we are on a spiritual ladder and knew how much I could handle in the process. It knew everything! Every time I fell asleep, *it* woke me up with the loud noise of horns and cymbals fanfare. I was in a circus! Making me hear the sounds of people puking was telling me to go throw up when it was needed!

There was not a single moment I was not aware and awake! And *it* made sure that I stayed *awake* too. After all, I did pray to the spirit of the plant before starting the ceremony, "If I can take it, (the lessons) give it all to me."

In the middle of all my early journeys with ayahuasca, the thought of, "Why the heck did I put myself into such a thing?" always crept in. I was not feeling good at all; I felt nauseous most of the time. I felt like all of my internal organs, and my eyeballs were going to be expelled with the puking, and the loud sounds of the circus music kept me from going back to unconsciousness. It needed me to be and kept me awake at all times. I bow to the intelligence of ayahuasca that helped me awaken and has kept me awake ever since.

All ayahuasca teachings were tough. No part of the healing was spared. I went (or was it my mind?) through all the possible human emotions one after another: cold, thirst, hunger, pain, despair, abandonment, shame, guilt, weakness, *fear*, greed, etc. I "saw" and experienced all my fears, starting as a child and going through adulthood – a fear I gladly died to in more than one session.

Fear is the hardest thing for everyone to overcome. I felt like I was dying to my old self, my "human self," and my beliefs and an illusory world. I was dying at each ceremony, again and again. Each time after that, I came back for more until my mind was cleansed and reconstructed as it should have always been – or until there was nothing left to die from.

What comes after all of this is a Self that stands tall and unblemished, unencumbered by illusion and falsity taught in this lifetime and beyond. The emotional body is significantly healed and strengthened; it raises our immune system immensely. The most recent ceremony I went under, the whole left side of my body got fixed. It was like a three-hour body adjustment session with the plant medicine. It worked on my neck, shoulder, and jaw. I still can't figure out how it happened, but it did, and I was fully awake to witness the strength of its work. I have not had a cold or been sick for six years since I started working with this plant medicine.

I now have a stronger body and mind. I am a better mother, friend, coworker, and healer to myself and others. The lesser part with ayahuasca is the puking. It might be hard for some people. But we only puke out the bad stuff that needs to be evacuated.

Every morning after the ceremony was a brand-new beginning. A total rebirth occurs from the abyss of a dark night spent under the stars as a witness of the soul work well-done.

Everyone's experience is different; having no expectations before an ayahuasca ceremony is highly recommended. You will never know what to expect because it has an intelligence of its own. It is always a surprise. More is not necessarily better; it's all about how far you are on the spiritual path, how much can you take, and how deep into the rabbit hole you want to go. The choice of how many cups you can drink is yours to make. It can be spread over time, like ten years, if you wish so.

If you are considering rebirth or healing (it can be both), there are many ways to enhance your journeys and transform you truly. DMT is by far the most mind-blowing way to recode all of your broken mind and body wirings. Since the mind is tightly linked to your diseases and illnesses, it could be the help you need to experience. It may provide quick and profound relief to your mind or whatever you wish to transform in your life.

Rest assured, the Universe will guide you through it all. We are *never* alone. This kind of experience cannot be supported by pure scientific research yet; however, there are many books about DMT, and they all agree it is genuinely helping people from all walks of life. I used this help and experienced deep, profound change and transformation in my life and my being. No doubts – we need to die to this little "me and I."

One of my patients suffered from anxiety and has been on medication for twenty years; after one DMT session, he ditched his meds that same week. It's been two months now, and he is anxiety and medication free. True story.

PAST LIFE REGRESSION THERAPY (PLRT)

For those adept in past-life theory, PLRT merely is going backward in time to understand, heal, and move forward in time instead of staying stuck on just third steps. Most of us go from childhood to adolescence and get stuck in adulthood. What happened to Godhood? Man's true evolution is still barbaric, and most of us remain complacent in the stage of infancy. The enjoyment of the five senses is the stumbling block of all there is.

I learned to regress people who believe in this type of work. It is better if someone believes in this kind of work, but it still works if they don't. The person goes into deep relaxation (we can call it trance), and he/she is led to explore the past and retrieve damaging emotions/trauma at his/her roots. Relieving them can bring deep healing to the sufferers, who sometimes do not know why they live in terror of something they cannot explain.

The session can be lengthy, up to three or four hours and sometimes more. I ask many questions during the first intake meeting; then, we move into the induction to access theta brain waves, where all answers are. We can retrieve much information in just one session, and healing can be automatically achieved by going deep into the problem's roots

PLRT healed my fear of water by having a spontaneous past life regression where I clearly saw myself drowning. Another time, I saw myself living as a man in South America burdened by sadness, and the stories helped me understand the person I am today. These two experiences substantially impacted me and made me want to learn about past life regression therapy and use it on others to help them move along.

Going into past life is not always necessary for everyone to heal, but when we desire to do so, it can explain our present condition and help us move forward with closure and coming to terms with long-standing pain.

I had good results with one patient who had fibromyalgia. She went under the past life regression, and she confronted a situation that kept her in anger. Understanding the why and when about this deep anger she felt gave her new abilities to accept herself, move toward long-lasting healing, and eliminate her illness symptoms.

7

FOUR PROVEN AND SUCCESSFUL METHODS I USE TO TREAT FM

ACUPUNCTURE TO THE RESCUE

I became adept with acupuncture in 1996 after talking to my friend TJ, who swore by it. I remember my deep interest in healing naturally and holistically, so this method was very attractive. I went to school for three years, studying the whole acupuncture program, including Chinese herbs. After practicing for twenty-one years, I am sure that this ancient healing system is truly a life savior for humanity.

Over the last twenty years, it has become more popular and accepted as an adjunct treatment or preventative medicine. Its early discovery five thousand years ago originated in China, and medical researchers keep improving and adding studies to understand better what it can do for the human body.

In terms of a good prognosis, the treatments need to be recurrent over time to create a full healing effect. The earlier the problem is detected, the more efficient acupuncture can be. I have had patients with debilitating health problems due to chemotherapy or painful conditions recover by using acupuncture.

Acupuncture consists of the insertion of fine needles at specific points along distributed meridians. Each meridian hosts an organ from head to toe. Ancient emperors of China used it. The ancient documents are still relevant to the procedure today, known as *The Yellow Emperor's Classic of Internal Medicine*, dating back to about 100 BC.

Acupuncture practice is an observation of the relation, interrelation, and communication between bodily organs and their interdependency, just like with humans. (As above, so below: the internal will reflect the external is the kind of relation I mean). It is also known with regard to the five elements: earth, water, metal, wood, and fire. The theory states that all of these elements are connected, and each element has a relationship with the others. Through understanding yin/yang theory, hot and cold pertaining to external invasion or internal body state, full or hollow organs, dryness versus dampness, etc., we can work with what is ailing a body. With keen external examination, we can understand the reflection of internal patterns of disease on the outside.

History indicates that ancient sages received profound visions while in meditation within nature. The ebb and flow of the body can be compared with nature at work; our bodies, indeed, are intricately connected with Mother Nature. In the earlier days in ancient China, stone, bones, and bamboo were the only tools they had to use in the practice of acupuncture. Today, we use needles made of stainless steel, making acupuncture safe and practical because the needles are single-use and discarded.

We can use acupuncture as preventative medicine. Since the WHO recognized acupuncture as an effective way to treat over fifteen medical conditions, it is covered by insurance companies, mainly for painful conditions. Medicare now accepts and covers acupuncture under certain restrictions. It is also covered by the Veterans Association to treat PTSD.

In my experience, acupuncture is useful for everything and everybody. I have never encountered any problem with this form of healing – it is safe and effective. In China and Vietnam, acupuncture can be performed daily, but here in America, it is commonly applied twice or once per week for patients. It is useful for treating all sorts of pain, insomnia, nervous system disorders, respiratory disorders, headaches, FM, hormonal problems, libido issues, digestion problems, anxiety, depression, the flu, lung disorders, paralysis, traumas, and more.

BIORESONANCE MEDICINE

We are energy. In this context, energy means an area or open space, as an operative field or visual field, which is not necessarily visible to the untrained eyes. Science recently shed light on the electromagnetic field generated by all living cells. We also possess a field called the biofield or etheric field pattern, a more subtle field emanating and pulsing life that we can detect and treat. It is our subtle energy field.

The electromagnetic field provides a link between the etheric body and the nervous system. Our nervous system is one of the most complex and intricate systems in our body and nature itself.

In spiritual science, when we fix the biofield surrounding our body first, health will ensue. Because this electromagnetic field can be seen as our Self, and to my knowledge and experience, in turn, influences our whole health and well-being greatly.

Sensitiv Imago scans/ bioresonance therapy is a device I successfully use in my practice to help people with FM. It allows the person to see the scanning on a screen and determine what heavy metals, toxins, parasites, viruses, and bacteria are in their body system and what food is causing an allergic reaction.

The Sentiv Imago 500 from Ukraine is a complete healing system and scanning device used around the world. Using it is such a great help in safely scanning my patients to treat them with the most efficient vibrational and energetic medicine. The device scans, treats, and diagnosis the body altogether with 96 percent accuracy by treating the energetic field. The body is supplied with the perfect frequency for the work: detoxing, restoring, and healing. Its main functions are:

- Detecting the Presence of viruses, parasites, and bacteria, including their localization and the level of harmful effects on the patient

- Diagnosing the disease and the extent of its development

- Analyzing all systems of organs, blood, and functional and structural changes

- Finding chemicals, toxins, and heavy metals present in the body

- Treating the body with bioresonance therapy

- Eliminating pain

I like to make my patients conscious of their breath at all times. Breathing regulates the mind and, in turn, relaxes the body.

I became a kundalini yoga instructor in 2000. Little by little, all the means and knowledge to first experience and then understanding how to enhance our beings were gathered together for me to advance in this quest, and now, I invite you to ignite the spark of walking the path.

Life is yoga itself. Its definition is "union with God (by many means)" – in body, mind, and spirit. Most people see it in the West as a form of poses and exercises that can unite us with our higher Self. We experience personal wellness and deep calmness. In the West, people think and practice mainly hatha yoga (yoga of the body). However, there are also other forms of yoga whose names we might not be familiar with.

Yoga can be taken seriously by practicing its deeper forms to understand the meaning of "union with God." It includes *pranayama* (breathing) and deep observance of spiritual qualities, such as celibacy, vegetarian food intake, ethical standards or moral conducts, nonviolence, non-attachments, and not stealing. As you can see, real yoga is not a trend. It is a way of life and conscious control over our human tendencies to attain the divine union.

Those who practice hatha yoga know that being light is a necessity while doing the exercises. And for the love of yoga, they had to learn to eat better as well. Some of them became vegetarian or vegan because of it. Taking up yoga will be a great ally in your search for health or truth. As this food choice is more sattvic in nature, it will provide feelings of wholeness and heal your body and mind. Yoga with *qigong* exercises is one of my favorite recommendations. Because both practices are fantastic for forming healthy habits and slowing down the mind, you will make better diet choices before exercising.

Karma Yoga

Karma yoga is the path of service with selfless action and assisting others in experiencing the divine in all.

Bhakti Yoga

This is a way to express our love for God through devotional rituals, prayers, devotional chanting, singing the names of God, and ceremony. I underwent training in India with a devotional fire ceremony call *yagya*. It is a fire of devotion that cleanses the human tendencies accumulated over many lives and worships the divine with sacred fire and Vedic mantras. I met a master who willingly taught me this practice, which I now implement regularly.

Jnani Yoga

This is the path of intellect and wisdom, including studying sacred texts, intellectual discussion, philosophical and spiritual debates, and introspection – all as a path of awakening.

Raja Yoga

Also known as the Royal Path, this consists of practicing all paths mentioned previously: physical, service, devotion, and intellect.

Yoga has different styles in different schools and teachers, but the traditional teachings remain the same. Don't worry; all of that does not need to be activated at the same time. The path will unfold gradually and naturally without any conscious effort or sacrifice from the seeker. Everything takes time, patience, and endurance. Accept and love exactly where you are and proceed from that idea.

8

HEALING WITH THE HELP OF OUR SPIRIT

S piritual growth is a lifetime of dedicated work. It is not an easy task and should be cultivated daily; it is cumulative, and the dividend is more than worthwhile. In all honesty, it is not for the faint of heart, nor is it for the people who have a hard time concentrating or taking potent stimulants or for lukewarm-hearted people who think of it as a trend. It is long and arduous. It can seem lonely and boring (only at the beginning) for many people because they feel their life will be restricted somehow. That's so far from the truth. If it hasn't taunted you yet to embark on such a journey, in my opinion, it means you have not suffered enough, or your spiritual maturity has not yet begun. Therefore, you will not (or might not) look for such a remedy to your life.

Unless a person is affected by fibromyalgia, my viewpoint remains the same. To my knowledge, it is possible to be free from fibromyalgia because freedom starts by freeing the mind of old programming, decades of false beliefs, and thoughts that true health and healing are something outside of ourselves. If you are physically able and sane enough to step in and do the spiritual work with little restrictions, the possibility of healing will be unsurpassed. But it depends on your invested effort.

If we can find the brighter side of any situation and extract only the positive, it will greatly reduce its gravity, at least by 50 percent. It starts with mind work first, and then, with eagerness and determination, you can move forward to resolve it with all that you've got by diving into spiritual work.

Unfortunately, I meet patients with only the desire to get better, but just desire is not enough; I always try to gently push them forward, enticing them with health and happiness for harnessing. Because of the constant coaching and repetition that I supply them with, they see great results. The percentage of people who sincerely work for their true healing is not a big one. We are just so caught up with the mind taking us to so many places it is hard for anyone to see the trees in the forest. It does take someone who is spiritually mature or can see that we are just living a life of recurring pain and suffering to want to change. It is not easy to do it by yourself than by doing it with someone who walks the walk. We always need teachers along the path. We can take the horse to the water; the rest is his doing.

Developing a real sense of Self is necessary for this endeavor – not a Self that can be discouraged as soon as the wind changes its direction, someone says something, or you read something that sets you back on the internet. All resolution goes out the window. That is a weak and fluctuating mind – little can be achieved with this kind of mentality.

We all have a Self we show to the world and people in our daily lives, and many people don't even know who their true Self is. Instead, they mistake their personality for their true Self. I am talking about the authentic Self: an unchanging Self or deep Presence within us. If we feel hurt, changeable, or moody, that is not the Self; it's ego or personality that is unstable and changeable.

Your deeper Self can be developed with sincere introspection and in silence. It will help you be more observant and aware at all times. It is a place where we can heal and be at peace forever. Therefore, going into meditation every day is so important, as it will show you what your true Self is and, from a place of silence, rearrange and reorganize everything in your life.

The Self can only show up when we are deep in stillness and silence. When we are immobile and aware, the connection with our divine Self can happen. We finally drop the analyzing mind/ego and acknowledge something bigger and more significant than this little body. Our receptivity is now received by the above, and because we are listening in stillness, the reward shows up. It's a giving thing. "You stay still and let me do the work for you!" "Man know Thyself!" How hard could it be?

Our bodies were created for health and healthy enjoyment. Our minds are for creating and surrounding ourselves with beauty. Getting lost in the gross illusion world and chasing the familiar thrill without preparing for the exit leaves us depleted to complete our life. After overusing this body, we weaken our nervous system, and we no longer effectively perform long sitting because the body feels restless. Meditate and raise the consciousness for a higher understanding of the power within. God and health are *one* and the *same.*

The key to a heightened ability to feel everything is being present and listening to the Self silently. The Universe converses with us through silence. All the solutions we seek in life come to us with direct interaction with the universal intelligence. Do not think *it* cannot hear us; *we* cannot hear it.

Once the Presence is firmly established within us, it will remain there forever. It accumulates and grows more and more over time. It is the only treasure to be discovered. We cannot treat this achievement of a lifetime too cheaply. Thinking of money, time, and energy as obstacles are bad excuses. Give all that you have – that may be even our well-being and comfort, as hard as it may sound. It is the Almighty Creator we are talking about, after all – more important than a president or a pope. It's our alpha and our omega.

Let me know how much you are willing to give in exchange for the gift of perfect bliss and union with Self, Presence, and God. Give everything you have if it takes that. The feeling of the Love/ God we receive in return is incomparable to anything you will ever experience in this dimension.

In the ancient past, people could only overcome one or two major hurdles in one lifetime. Today, with new waves of cosmic blessings entering the earth, we can directly shoot straight to the High Consciousness CEO. We can do all of that in one lifetime if we want to. Forget about limitations; all it takes is a firm determination to conquer our minds.

We can burn karma in the fire of our devotion. Just fix your mind on God's name; everything will be taken care of. By incessantly glorifying His/ Her name, we will become that perfection in time. We are redefining ourselves not as a human but as one with God. That is what Jesus came to teach.

The power of our consciousness can pierce the veil of separation of *us* and the almighty God, like a laser beam cutting through a thick, earthy crust before revealing a flawless diamond. We are diamonds in the rough, waiting to uncover our magnificent shine. The work required for this weighs on us to achieve this priceless gift.

I was born in a Buddhist country and raised as a Christian Catholic. My children's father is a Jew, and I practice Vedantic philosophy (from India).

So, in the next sentence from Jesus, I do not make a religious statement, but I will use these words of our Master Jesus to get the point across:

"If anyone would come after me, let him deny himself and take up his cross and follow me. For whoever would save his life will lose it, but whoever loses his life for my sake will find it. For what will it profit a man if he gains the whole world and forfeits his soul?"

Jesus spoke in subtle ways that were hard for someone who was not enlightened to understand. His consciousness was *one* with God at all times; he was a fully realized God being walking on this earth two thousand years ago. But He (with all due respect) was our human brother as well. He understood our potential as gods. He saw our unmanifested Self suffocated and gasping for air. He understood the need for humans to die to their egoic mind and came to deliver a powerful message to mankind: "Thou are God." Was he heard? By some, but not by all.

"Let him deny himself" means, in layman's terms, "Children of God, let go of the ego." Kill it with your spiritual effort day after day, moment after moment, for my sake. He was never in the egoic mind. He was one with God; he spoke from his God Self.

We cannot realize the Supreme Self with a mind built by ego and personality only. It is the perennial wall of separation between man and God. He never meant for us to follow him blindly like sheep. How good is it for Jesus to have blind follower's incapable of choosing from their own free will? We were not meant to understand his messages literally word for word but to understand the subtle *spirit* behind his words. His message was for us to understand the *work* it takes to reach the *one* supreme consciousness He was with "and that *we* can do it too," He said.

Living only to enhance our life physically or gain riches by accumulation is a trap to the spirit. Our God-Self needs to be rediscovered and sublimated by our effort. "Taking up his cross" means *accepting* what is in our life right now with *no* complaints, bowing our heads, being like little children carried by a pure heart, and working hard on ourselves to be reborn into the grandeur of our oneness with God's power in this life, *now* – not when we die!

Please, don't wait to die to see God and heaven because we will miss the great purpose of this lifetime. This work is about going above and beyond all earthly illusions and religious teachings with all our mighty being (body, mind, suffering, and pain) to transcend this human mind, fulfill our godly duties, and grow spiritually. Don't delay.

We are living a life that does not offer all of the entirety we were supposed to receive. We made the choices based on incomplete knowledge passed down from generation to generation and were steeped in profound ignorance of Self. This statement is not a condemnation of it, of course. Everything unfolded as it should, but now, the wake-up call has rung to remind us the time is due. We have grown way past the previous dark age; are we going to roll over still, choose to stay asleep, and behave like sheep? Are we just designed for an un-awakened life, wasting time and time again, lifetime after lifetime?

Let's *wake up*, powerful creators that we are! Stop being the actors in this scary movie. Recall that our sovereignty has been sent through the master of many ages time and time again as a reminder. No, we don't have to be super religious, have thirty years of experience as a meditator, or live in India under the supervision of a guru (even though that idea is excellent if you want to and can do it). Your choice to realize your true Self is waiting for a different chapter to be created. Just be mindful of the necessary basic things: a laser focus, an unflinching willingness, a deep sincerity, and a yearning to know the truth and believe the Universe will assist you in that endeavor and make it possible for you to attain.

I observed most of my patients only wanting to be well but not putting in real effort to grow. They kept coming back. True to myself, I probed them and triggered them with little hints, but I could not get to the deepest part of them due to a lack of time and appropriate circumstances. In truth, they just wanted a fix. "The primary healer is not doing her job," they said. I'm thinking, "What can I do? I am only secondary to their healing."

Don't ignore a treasure of happiness by remaining numb and living your life without wondering the real reason for your existence. True self-awakening or realization of who we are will change the way we think of ourselves and others. Because everything is always related to our Self, big or small, our inner world will reflect us how fulfilled, sad, or happy we are. God is a field of infinite energetic potential, a feeling of harmony, and perfect balance.

There are many treatments offered out there. We can bring this body and mind from unbalance to a perfect state of harmony, which will propel us to step up into another level of life with more achievements. The strong foundation of health can be based on body repair or readjustment, mind work, and spiritual endeavor.

Repairing only the body, which is a long term goal, is just a lopsided and shortsighted decision. My days of treating symptoms served their time. I bow to all teachers who brought me to this point. I now know there is more to life than we ever could think of; health is just a start. I awoke myself first, and now I come to help you awaken if you choose so. One size treatment does not fit all, but the Self is the same for us *all*. The body can be forgiving with a straight mindset, and the Universe is benevolent toward its creatures.

Therefore, I call this the work of a lifetime. We are bombarded with myriad things to accomplish in life. We could be lost in a labyrinth of earthly duties while forgetting the real goal. The complete amnesia sets in. As spiritual beings, we will be here for another twenty, thirty, or forty years. Then *what?* How can amassing more stuff help us on Exodus Day?

Leo Tolstoy said, "Wisdom is to know what is the meaning of life and to follow it." Because it takes time and energy, many toiled their entire lives to build massive wealth, homes, and businesses. What happens when it is over? The mind becomes too stiff and brittle to do anything new. Blood slows down. The body is not getting any younger. The energy to pursue knowledge and truth isn't present. "God who? What's that?"

I feel I am more of a behind-the-scenes person – the kid who used to be always in the back of the classroom entirely at ease with being invisible to the world. I am captivated by the weird things – the more mysterious, the better. Whether you call it bending reality or going through a wormhole, writing about fibromyalgia and God is kind of a hot subject to me.

We are all kids (in the eyes of the cosmic Universe, we are kids) living a dream. We don't know squat until we are ready to learn fearlessly – not only from the world as we see it but also from the Great Unknown –and to discover something so unbelievably grand that we can fall madly in love with all our heart night and day, every day, again and again until the end. This love, I know, never feels old, never demands anything of us, and never tarnishes. It just keeps growing vastly. We can only exhale pure bliss.

"People of the land!" We can still enjoy all in this life and, at the same time, move our feet to a higher goal. Life will taste so much sweeter, and more beauty will be present to adorn your eyes. We do not see the world as it is; *we* see it as *we* are. Buddha said that once upon a time, and it still rings true.

We are a part of the grand solution by birthing a new healthy network of pure minds. We do it because our children will also inherit a healthy legacy with spiritual treasures to enjoy. The solution to perfect health and enjoyment of life is for *us* alone to decide which way to go. The choice is for each person to make.

I shared with you what we can do and how to cross over the boundaries of our seemingly secured life and the limited mind. Acupuncture, PLRT, DMT-5 MEO DMT – it all might sound strange to you, but that's okay. It sounded weird to me when I first started my journey. I came into this one existence strangely organized by the Universe, and until I started writing this book, I felt a voice inside me for years, saying, "Share what you have learned. Write this book".! Those are fast but safe methods.

9

OBSTACLES

During this effort of building a spiritual body and a healthy mind, which will render you whole, there will be many obstacles. The first obstacle is the mind. The mind is very cunning and smart. The Antichrist could be your mind; no need to look on the outside. The enemy is within.

If, along the way of your spiritual practice, you think you fell off track because something disturbing happened, just get back on the horse ASAP and try not to feel sorry for yourself for more than two days; take your mind off it and fix it firmly on your chosen deity. I'm not trying to be insensitive; it's just your positive vibrations you have started to build need to stay high, and the longer you pity yourself, the deeper you fall back into a lower frequency and the harder it is to go back up. The fact is that the more we give in to our weakness, the more it stays.

I give you this advice with love. If you tend to whine or feel sorry for yourself easily: please take a deep breath and change your mind's track – it will not be helping you. It might not be easy at first, and it might even feel very uncomfortable – especially if you have to learn about meditation and being still, for example. One of the main reasons you can't stay still is because your mind is racing all the time toward an outcome far in the future. The body and the mind need to even out with each other; if the mind becomes calm, the body will also. Staying in the present will take you there. For the visualization part, if you are a left-brain thinker, you might get frustrated. If this is the case, just say out loud what you are imagining/visualizing or look at something that is soul-elevating. As time goes by and you keep going and doing, something will give in for the better, and the new *you* will emerge.

Life-altering change takes effort. I'm not talking about superficial change, like patching and fixing your pains; continuing to chase your tail will get old, and it will take you nowhere. We doctors will keep seeing you, again and again, year after year, listening to your unresolved complaints. It does not make us feel better.

Even though I was raised in a religion, I found no real depth to my prayer words when I started to pray again at twenty-three. All of it was lip-synching; it was empty of meanings and sincerity. I had no clear visions of what I was to do to earn my living. I was confused between what I felt and what I was taught.

My personal feelings were the only things that guided me; those were real and guiding light.

For those who have not yet developed a certain sense of knowing their spiritual Self, it might be challenging at the beginning. Just practice engaging the other side of your brain, where all abstract ideas, spiritual concepts, arts, languages, and intuitions live. It's about engaging your whole brain; indeed, two sides of the brain working together in collaboration are better than just one side.

If those things are difficult for you to grasp, don't be discouraged. Give them a try to train your mind day by day. If we can go to the gym and train the body to grow muscles and stay fit, we can do the same thing to tame the mind. Like a wild horse, it needs to be controlled. In doing so, you will harness the power to reshape your health and your entire future in a short time.

The important truth to keep in mind is that no one can do this *work* for you. When it comes to chronic health issues, there is *no* savior outside of yourself. And as far as I am concerned, I love Him too, but Jesus is not coming back to save us. As harsh as it may sound, for health, happiness, and ascension, you are indeed the only one to do it – by yourself, for yourself.

Distractions are many in this world, and they might be significant obstacles: people, friends, or family members who aren't supportive of this kind of work. We may feel like we want to belong with them and not feel so different or labeled. Just know that they might not be there for you when you need them, or they may only show up when your life is on the up but not if it is going down. Be firm with your practice and loyal to your Self – it is your only true friend in this life and the afterlife.

Keep your practice for yourself, or share it only with people who support you and celebrate your desire to raise your consciousness. Keep the practice at the same time and place; do not waver or change. If it is 6:00 a.m. or 10:00 p.m., stay on the program.

I keep a spiritual program daily and recourse with masters/gurus in India when I feel I need inspiration. Sometimes, being with enlightened people helps us stay on the path and gives us a little boost to carry on the work.

Excuses to not to meditate will be created by the (old) mind every day, don't give in, after a while when, positive feelings (your spirit) start to set in, you will feel more inclined to resume your spiritual practice, there will be more eagerness or even excitement about it, this is a good sign that you are more aligned with your divine nature.

10

MY WISH FOR YOU

"In the Fullness of the 'Presence' is the love that you require! In the Fullness of the 'Presence' are the things that you desire!"

— MASTER ST. GERMAIN

STEPS OF THE PROCESS

• If you think you can do this on your own, please do it. Otherwise, you could find a good holistic practitioner doctor/spiritual counselor you can trust to help in the process of detoxification.

• Remove clutter from your mind by going to the root and eliminate past baggage, negative beliefs, and traumas with digging works.

• Pick up some form of spiritual yoga and/or *qigong* or tai chi practice (these build life force, *qi, prana*).

• Detoxify the body from parasites, flukes, bacteria, mold, fungus, etc.

• Do the liver gall bladder flush.

• Consider Implementing a balanced nutrition program.

• Practice some form of meditation daily, such as silent meditation, breathing meditation, chakra meditation, or walking meditation, as silence reconnects you with the Source.

• As a sub-meditation, practice silent inquiries and deep introspection.

• Spend time in nature and connect with it.

• Find therapies that suit your body and mind.

• Find a genuine guru if you feel spiritually inclined.

Everything happening to us in life is the same for everyone; it comes in different shapes, colors, countries, themes, languages, feelings of joy, and pain and disease sensations. For the most part, we do all experience the same feelings and emotions of love or hate. We all need to eat and sleep; we are the same at the core. All our basic needs are the same for everyone. The common work that could be is we need to find the life remedies to our ills. The list I proposed could be just ideas to consider; you can find other avenues to get rid of your pain and sickness, of course. Many people will only accept it and do nothing and just drift, and still, life, somehow, will manage to take us back "home" one day, in time, slowly, no matter how long it takes. Because the only place we are all going is the home of Spirits. We can choose to do it fully awakened and healthy in this body this time, of course. The choice is ours.

I'm not so sure you want a return ticket.

Many possibilities make a person feel he/she cannot do the work. It could be "I don't believe in this stuff," "Don't complicate my life. I will give it to someone else so they can tell me what to do of my fibromyalgia," "I am too busy with my life" "It costs too much of my time and money," "I prefer to live with my sickness," or "It's cozier if I choose to stay asleep." I am sure there are many reasons.

But I say that is all ignorant ego talk. I assure you the Self wants itself to be known and revealed. Its magnificent wisdom knows that it is "Itself" living the pain and going through sufferings. An un-awakened person is devoid of this vision of urgency to raise his/her consciousness to meet with his/her higher destiny. His/her shadow blindly leads him/her to the grave.

Because the mortal flesh and truest spiritual intelligence are not supported by all the Cosmic Life forces necessary to sublimate them, the body template is dying from a form of slow suicide, and it grows ugly in the process. Nothing will be spared: the sad and tired look shows after fifty, grim bitterness and a loveless life read on the lips (only observation from my training in acupuncture), the absence of spirit shows in lusterless eyes. The health state will be in jeopardy because the spirit *is* everything. It's the true health of a body, the beauty of a face, the grace in our movement, the intelligence in our heart. Nothing truly beautiful comes from the body acting alone.

Through my ayahuasca visions, I was allowed to see how unconsciously burdened we all are, living daily with untold sufferings of many kinds (even aside from the seven capital sins). But what was most disturbing to me was the vision of all souls being bound and silenced, unable to get out in this world and anchor the true light in this dimension. I felt untold sorrows go through my heart. I melted in sorrow. After that, my life could never be the same as it had been. The change was permanent.

As I was waking up to my tardiness to do the true work myself, I was shown a vision from my third eye, an untold story of humans living in the deep ignorance of who *we* are: true living Gods in a deep sleep. I felt so contrite that night. I wanted to bring a small contribution to this world to help you wake up too and believe not in sickness or diseases, but in the mighty power within us. Think of yourself not as powerless "sinners" but as truth, light, and love. Then apply this vision to everybody else around you.

This life is meant for us to awaken and seize all opportunities with the determination and mighty heart of a true soldier for truth. Speak it, live it, and be *one* with *it*. You are not any form of sickness – never have been, never will be.

When it is appropriate, choose feelings versus thinking, silence versus noise, stillness versus movement, and acceptance versus judgment; become a hollow flute that the wind of heaven can dance through and create beautiful sounds with, blessing this earth with your Presence.

This world, as it appears, is seductive, tempting, and captivating. Like the Medusa, it will transform us into stone if we look at it for too long. This world of three-dimensional matrixes is thick and pulling us in so fast every second. Unfortunately, most can't even realize for a second that it is not real. The moment we awaken, self-actualize, and see our true nature, we can be changed quickly for the best outcome. *The consciousness* of who we are is the remedy to every ill that plagues us today.

We are all divine children lost in a long-forgotten past, unable to find our way "home" to our true Self. We can be compared as hopeless mendicants going from place to place like poor beggars, with nothing to eat or wear, running amok and losing our minds altogether, creating sickness and pain for one another. "What an asylum this world is," a mother saint of India (Anandayi Maa) said – and I concur with her now after twenty-four cups of DMT (and not a saint yet). This world is a place where men/Gods lose their minds and can't remember a thing!

The remedy for awakening is fixing your mind on the Creator with a sacred mantra at all times. *This* is perennial – changing the ongoing mind always disturbed by thoughts. Make it calm and clear. In time, with practice, like Superman, you will be able to do two or three things simultaneously, such as driving and saying your mantra. Being in meditation all the time and saying the mantra as you deal with the world is essential for clearing and calming. Seeing as God in action is like the breathless lotus flower with its roots deep in the mud (the world), and its head turned to the sun (light).

The mantra sound is God Himself (or Herself, if you wish to picture God like that). Your mind should always be like that: focused on the prize. And *that* which you think *will* manifest – I can guarantee you. Give it time and practice, practice, practice. This Presence will blow your little mind away! It will become everything you wish for. It is the mother and the Father at the same time, the true unconditional healer and strength you can rely on. It will be there for you more than your family and friends. It will prepare the day and even your vacation for you. It will take care of your children and help you cope with it all. It will provide for your every need. It will take the load off your shoulders. It is nearer than near; it is awaiting *you*. Fall in love with your Self, and the world will be in love with *you*.

People suffering from fibromyalgia, if you believe in God and not in the power within your Self, it will defeat the purpose of coming to experience this life in the body you possess right now. You have chosen this seemingly complicated path of health even if you don't remember. If you chose this path, you did so because you are that strong as a soul and because you knew you could do it. The challenge right now is to go over the bumpy road that feels real and unsurmountable, but it is for you to pick up. You don't have to do it all alone. Call on your mighty Self, your God-given power, to rise and assist you in this transformation at hand. Wake up! It's just a dream.

My wish for you is incommensurable. Doing this work is the highest work of humankind – and the hardest. Perfect yourself in your mind and heart to become *one* with Self and be the best godly human you can be.

May the light be with you in everything you do, and may the perfect decision to improve your Self finds you.

ACKNOWLEDGMENTS

A huge thanks to all my spiritual teachers who shared their priceless love and pointed the way for us to know Self and beyond: Thanks to Guruma Rokmani and Guru Rajneesh Rishi, Shni Dev, Sri Babaji of the Himalayas, Master Jesus, Saint Germain, Amrita Nandamayi Ma, Shree Maa, Sri Tatatha, Aghoreshwar Bhagwan Ramji, Yogi Bhajan, and Osho.

Thanks to my mother, Jeanette, who taught me unconditional love and somehow imparted in me not to attach myself to anything. Thanks to all my family members, especially my sisters, Solange Nguyen Van Binh and Monique Nguyen Van Binh, and Suzanne Marechal, for the work you did while growing up and my precious children, Jos and Caden Brown.

Thanks to all my friends who delighted my existence with countless moments of joy and sharing. Thanks to my dear friends Martha Montes De Oca, Ernesto Beltre, Gloria, and Scott Ellis for their support and friendship over all these years. Warm thanks to all my patients, past and present; I was honored to be a part of your healing journey.

Thanks to Jay A. Nielsen, my partner, who inspired me to move ahead and get this book in writing, for his encouraging support.

A million grateful thanks to the great Creator, the One and Only, the One in Many, the force behind our existence.

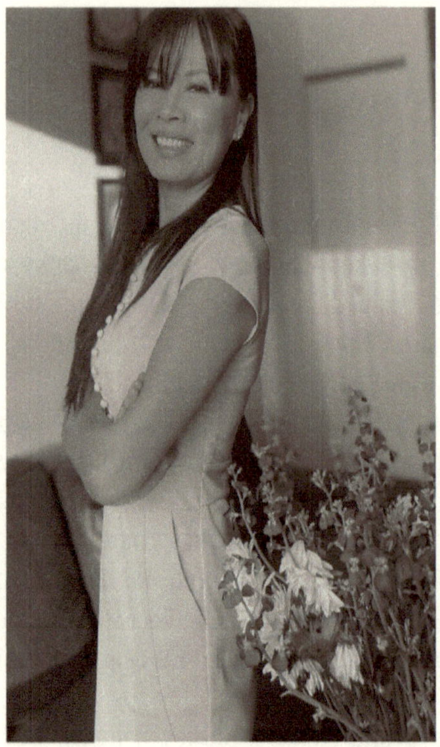

Dr. Nicole Nguyen Van Binh was born in Saigon, Vietnam, in 1962. She was raised in France from the age of eight by Catholic nuns. She developed most of her spiritual nature under this strict education, which left her with more questions than answers. She went through a traditional French school system until the age of eighteen.

Having no means to pursue higher education and no job prospects in France, her life at nineteen put her on a train with twenty dollars in her pocket, heading to Geneva, Switzerland. She quickly found a job handling the front desk of a sporting club. She connected well with the path of least resistance. She was floating with no place or home to anchor her, but everything felt all right to her.

In her early adult life, she followed her dream to learn English and traveled the world. At the same time, she was drawn by a deeper search of who she was and why she was here in this life.

Having wide-open eyes and ants in her pants, she jumped on all opportunities to travel, and the African continent was her home for another five years, living off whatever jobs she could land to meet her living expenses. Some would see that as not being rooted, but she wanted as many experiences as she could fit in before reaching thirty. The constant curiosity and fearlessness in discovery enticed her to travel the world; a carrier and family were not on her priority list. There would be time for this later. She was then drawn to India, Asia, South America, and all the spiritual places she could visit and learn from.

Her training was not in the pursuit of higher education. She felt she was supposed to accumulate all of her learning through life in every way presented to her, good or bad.

When she landed in Miami in 1994, it was time to start working in the system. She wanted to perform in a domain that would give her the freedom to think and exist with few restrictions. She became an LMT and then was led to the world of healing. She is presently a diplomate in acupuncture and Chinese medicine and a mother to two beautiful ten-year-old twin boys. Her practice, anchored in southern Miami, Florida, provides health and spiritual counseling, acupuncture and Chinese medicine, energetic medicine, cranial sacral therapy, body talk, and past life regression hypnosis. She is a facilitator for DMT and consciousness.

ABOUT DIFFERENCE PRESS

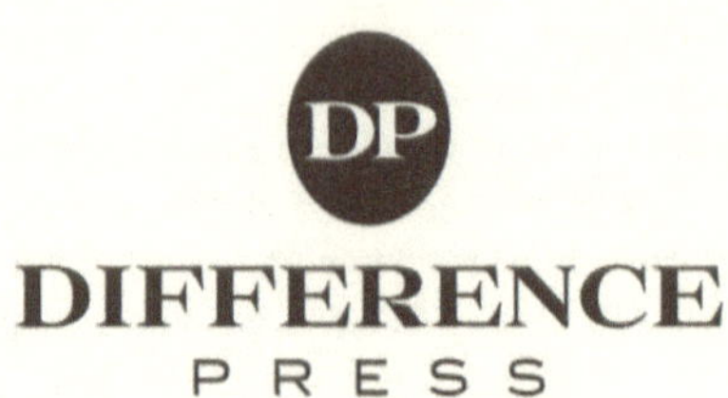

Difference Press is the exclusive publishing arm of The Author Incubator, an educational company for entrepreneurs – including life coaches, healers, consultants, and community leaders – looking for a comprehensive solution to get their books written, published, and promoted. Its founder, Dr. Angela Lauria, has been bringing hundreds of authors-in-transformation's literary ventures since 1994.

A boutique-style self-publishing service for clients of The Author Incubator, Difference Press boasts a fair and easy-to-understand profit structure, low-priced author copies, and author-friendly contract terms. Most importantly, all of our #incubatedauthors maintain ownership of their copyright at all times.

LET'S START A MOVEMENT WITH YOUR MESSAGE

In a market where hundreds of thousands of books are published every year and are never heard from again, The Author Incubator is different. Not only do all Difference Press books reach Amazon bestseller status, but all of our authors are actively changing lives and making a difference.

Since launching in 2013, we've served over 500 authors who came to us with an idea for a book and were able to write it and get it self-published in less than six months. In addition, more than 100 of those books were picked up by traditional publishers and are now available in bookstores. We do this by selecting the highest quality and highest potential applicants for our future programs.

Our program doesn't only teach you how to write a book – our team of coaches, developmental editors, copy editors, art directors, and marketing experts incubate you from having a book idea to being a published, bestselling author, ensuring that the book you create can actually make a difference in the world. Then we give you the training you need to use your book to make the difference in the world, or to create a business out of serving your readers.

ARE YOU READY TO MAKE A DIFFERENCE?

You've seen other people make a difference with a book. Now it's your turn. If you are ready to stop watching and start taking massive action, go to http://theauthorincubator.com/apply/.

"Yes, I'm ready!"